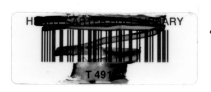

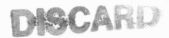

Hepatitis C
The Silent Killer

Carol Turkington

CB
CONTEMPORARY BOOKS

Library of Congress Cataloging-in-Publication Data

Turkington, Carol.
    Hepatitis C : the silent killer / Carol Turkington ; foreword by
Joseph B. McCormick and Susan Fisher-Hoch.
        p.   cm.
    Includes bibliographical references and index.
    ISBN 0-8092-2958-7
    1.   Hepatitis C—Popular works.   I.   Title.
RC848.H425T87   1998
616.3'623—dc21   97-53202
                                                       CIP

Interior design by Precision Graphics

Published by Contemporary Books
A division of NTC/Contemporary Publishing Group, Inc.
4255 West Touhy Avenue, Lincolnwood (Chicago), Illinois 60646-1975 U.S.A.
Printed in the United States of America
International Standard Book Number: 0-8092-2958-7
18   17   16   15   14   13   12   11   10   9   8   7   6   5   4   3   2   1

Also by Carol Turkington

The Brain Encyclopedia
The Encyclopedia of Deafness and Hearing Disorders
The Encyclopedia of Memory and Memory Disorders
The Hearing Loss Sourcebook
Home Health Guide to Poisons and Antidotes
The Hypericum Handbook
Making the Cold Less Common
Making the Prozac Decision: A Guide to Antidepressants
The Perimenopause Handbook
Poisons and Antidotes
Skin Deep: The Encyclopedia of Skin and Skin Disorders
Stress Management for Busy People

CONTENTS

The epidemic of hepatitis C now sweeping the world has been described as "the sleeping giant." In many communities particularly in developing countries, the hepatitis C epidemic equals or surpasses the epidemic of HIV. This means that in many places there are more people infected with hepatitis C and therefore more potential deaths from liver disease than HIV-infected people and deaths from AIDS. Somehow the hepatitis C virus has not gained public attention, and therefore the resources and scientific efforts to find treatment and vaccines are minute compared with the efforts that have been poured into research and treatment of AIDS. Hepatitis C is difficult to treat effectively and to prevent because, just like AIDS, hepatitis C is a chronic, persistent infection that has found a way to evade the defenses of the immune system. Effective vaccines are proving difficult to produce.

There is little information available to the general public as well as to those suffering from hepatitis C infection. As with AIDS, the knowledge that you are infected with this virus can be life shattering. Though the outcome is not as uniformly dire as with HIV infection, anyone who discovers that he or she is infected with the hepatitis C virus faces an uncertain future with all the fears attendant on the prospect of chronic, painful disease and possibly death. This knowledge can be devastating, and infected people need good advice and psychological support.

This book provides a wealth of information in clear, unambiguous language for those who wish to be educated about hepatitis C, for those wishing to know how to prevent acquiring the infection, as well as for those unfortunate enough to be infected by the hepatitis C virus. It is well organized and provides the full range of information required to understand the means of infection with the virus and to recognize risk factors that individuals might have experienced in the past. It will also help readers to seek, to understand, and ultimately to get a diagnosis for themselves or a loved one. For those individuals who have learned that they are infected, or for the families of such persons, there is information on treatment, long-term outlook, support groups, and other vital concerns. Some of the advice should help in facing complications with a positive, constructive attitude, and even in avoiding some of the worst consequences of the infection.

Though written for North America, this book is more broadly applicable, particularly in the developing world, where the largest burden of hepatitis C infection is found. Estimates of infection in the United States range from 1 to 2 percent. In the developing world, the number of apparently healthy people infected by the virus can be as high as 2 to 7 percent. This means that one out of every fifteen people you pass walking down the street may be infected with the hepatitis C virus! Estimates of the number of infected people who may develop chronic liver disease vary widely from 20 percent to as high as 80 percent. Seen as individuals with disrupted lives and families, even 1 percent represents widespread hardship, pain, and emotional and financial stress.

In the United States and other industrial countries, many hepatitis C infections resulted from infected blood supply before the virus test was available and from treatment of diseases like hemophilia with blood products. In stark contrast, most of the transmission of hepatitis C in developing countries continues to take place in hospitals and clinics. This is a fact that may shock many American readers, but a fact nonetheless. Unfortunately, staff in clinics and hospitals in poor or remote areas in the developing world often have poor education and training, and sometimes not even basic medical qualifications, a consequence of chronic poverty and overpopulation. In many countries there are traditional healers without formal training, or more often medical practitioners whose only qualifications are a piece of wood and some paint. These people use techniques such as injections and minor surgery, usually with minimal or no sterilization procedures. They have adopted the medical model of the West, that is, treatment of disease with injections, drips, and surgery. What they have not learned is that misuse of these powerful tools can spread infections, especially viruses. Efforts may be made to sterilize equipment between use, but successful sterilization can be difficult in a clinic without electricity, and often even without running water. Usually what we see is a bloodstained syringe soaking in tepid soapy water.

Then there is the matter of expense. The clinic will try to save money by reusing equipment, and at the same time is driven to prescribe injectable drugs, because they make more money than when they hand out pills. Among patients, there is widespread belief that injections are more "powerful" and "work faster" than pills. In some peri-urban clinics we studied in one country where we were working recently, we found that 82 percent of all patients had received an injection on that visit. Many of these people only complained of mild symptoms, such as headaches, feeling weak, or having vague pains in various parts of the body. We asked for blood samples as part of our study and found that more than 60 percent of them were infected with hepatitis C; that is, six out of every ten people who walked out through the clinic doors. And for all we know, the other four may have been infected during their visit that day!

We in the developed world share some responsibility for this growing tragedy through installation of western practices in conditions where they may not be safely practiced. For example, blood transfusions are common in developing countries. Children with malaria and women undergoing difficult childbirth often receive transfusions, and these may be lifesaving. The common belief that receiving blood gives you strength leads to the overuse of transfusions. The blood is usually screened for hepatitis B, less frequently for AIDS, but rarely for hepatitis C. Why? First, because the importance of hepatitis C is not appreciated, but second, and more important, because the patented kit that is used to screen for hepatitis C costs more per test than the local cost of a pack of blood. The pricing of these kits in large part reflects patent royalties.

All of us—particularly those with investments in the health industry—are making money out of the test. We need to press for some provision for pricing low enough to make the test accessible to those who need it most. If we do not, the soaring epidemic in the poorest parts of the world will return to haunt us. We will pay in terms of health, lost industrial output, and pain. We need to do something to remedy the situation now. If we allow this global epidemic to rage on unchecked, it will, like AIDS, continue to profoundly affect our own societies.

On a more positive note, there is much we can do. Education about hepatitis C, the consequences of infection, and means to prevent transmission are among the most important. Informing the public is what this book sets out to do. We hope that it brings support and some comfort to those already suffering and, because of the information and education it provides, helps to prevent many future infections. It is only by disseminating this kind of knowledge that we can stem the tide of the global epidemic.

Joseph B. McCormick, M.D.
Susan Fisher-Hoch, M.D.

ACKNOWLEDGMENTS

Inevitably, a book like this comes about not just in working with doctors and researchers, but in hearing from patients themselves who struggle mightily not just to survive, but to triumph over a disease such as hepatitis C. For this reason, I'd like to thank the countless numbers of people on the Internet who have shared their experiences.

A special thanks to Joe McCormick and Susan Fisher-Hoch for taking time from their busy labs in France to work with me on this book.

I'd also like to thank Alan Brownstein and the staff of the American Liver Foundation, the *Hepatitis C Newsletter*, the National Institute of Diabetes and Digestive Disorders and Kidney Diseases, the National Library of Medicine, and the medical libraries of the Hershey Medical Center, the University of Pennsylvania Medical Center, and the National Institutes of Health.

Finally, thanks to Susan Schwartz at NTC/Contemporary Publishing for her expert editorial guidance, Bert Holtje of James Peter Associates for valuable support, and, as always, Michael and Kara.

This book is dedicated with heartfelt gratitude
to the scientists and physicians around the
world who fight the never-ending battle against
infectious disease.

INTRODUCTION

It's a disease that affects one out of every sixty Americans, yet most people know almost nothing about hepatitis C. Although the virus that causes the disease was identified ten years ago as the most common reason for liver transplants, scientists still know very little even today about how it is transmitted or how to treat it. And while it is almost four times more common than the virus that causes acquired immunodeficiency syndrome (AIDS), hepatitis C goes largely unreported outside medical circles except for its occasional celebrity victims: singer Naomi Judd, the late TV newsman Frank Reynolds, and actor Jim Nabors. Baseball great Mickey Mantle's drinking habits got a lot of attention, but it was actually alcohol in combination with the hepatitis C virus that wiped out his liver.

What experts do know is that the U.S. death toll from hepatitis C is likely to double or triple, and right now there are few weapons to slow down the process. While an estimated four million Americans carry the microbe, hepatitis C is a "mystery virus" because it has few symptoms and can hide undetected in the body for years. In fact, some people who have the virus never develop liver disease, but about half those affected do eventually develop a chronic form of the infection that in time will destroy the liver, either by cirrhosis or cancer.

Scientists do know a few things about hepatitis C: It's a blood-borne virus that is hard to transmit during sex or childbirth. Drug abusers are the primary source of infection. But scientists have no idea where almost half its victims were infected. We also don't know why:

- *women respond better than men to interferon, the only drug treatment*
- *obese patients respond less well to interferon*
- *patients infected with only one major hepatitis C species do better than those with many different species*

- *Egypt has the highest infection rate—20 percent of military recruits (the otherwise young and healthy)*
- *hepatitis C virus (HCV) is more prevalent among heterosexual than homosexual men*

Based on extensive research and interviews with scientists and physicians, this book provides you with accurate information about the risks of this virus, what you need to know about hepatitis C, and what you can do to take control of your health. Assuming this responsibility means knowing what to fear and what not to fear, when to ask questions, and when to seek more information. *Hepatitis C* will offer you this much-needed information.

HEPATITIS C RESEARCH

A portion of the royalties from this book will be donated to the American Liver Foundation for hepatitis C research. Anyone who would care to donate money for research on hepatitis C may send contributions to:

American Liver Foundation
1425 Pompton
Cedar Grove, NJ 07009
(201) 256-2550

CHAPTER I

YOUR HEALTHY LIVER

Your liver is the largest internal organ in your body—and the most complex. It plays a vital role in regulating the processes that keep you alive and performs many complicated tasks that are essential to the proper functioning of the entire body. In fact, just about everything you swallow that is absorbed into the bloodstream eventually passes through the liver, a three-pound organ that looks a little like a football nestling behind the lower ribs on the right side of your abdomen.

This complex chemical laboratory is on the job twenty-four hours a day performing a wide range of duties involving regulation, metabolism, and detoxification. Among its functions, the liver:

- *processes and stores nutrients*
- *manufactures substances your body needs*
- *regulates the composition of the blood*
- *metabolizes nutrients, drugs, and other substances*
- *detoxifies and excretes harmful substances*

PURIFICATION

The liver cleans and purifies the blood supply, breaking down certain chemical substances in the blood. All the blood that leaves your stomach and intestines must pass through the liver before it goes to the rest of the body. The liver metabolizes alcohol to supply energy or to be deposited as fat. It deactivates a range of harmful drugs (such as nicotine) and helps the rest of your body, but your liver cells pay a high price for these services and may become severely damaged in the process.

At the same time, many beneficial medicines are activated, rather than inactivated, in the liver. This activation is necessary before these drugs can begin working.

The liver plays an important part in removing toxins produced inside the body as well, converting them to substances that are easily eliminated from the body. For example, your body normally produces a large amount of ammonia in the intestines as you digest your food. The liver changes this harmful ammonia into urea, a substance that is carried safely out of the body in the urine.

SYNTHESIS

The liver does more than break down harmful substances. It also produces helpful ones by taking simple building blocks and combining them into larger units. A kind of refinery, the liver processes nutrients from the digestive tract into forms that are easier for the body to use.

For example, the liver manufactures most of the proteins found in the blood. One protein, called albumin, combines with other substances and carries them to where they are needed in the body. Proteins necessary to stop bleeding are also manufactured in the liver. Your liver also produces another helpful substance—bile, a greenish-brown fluid containing cholesterol and bile acids that is important for digestion. Bile flows from the liver through the cystic duct to your gallbladder, where it is stored. It is eventually emptied into the duodenum, where it helps absorb fats through the lining of the small bowel into the bloodstream. The bile acids are then reabsorbed in the small intestine and cycled into the liver, to be used again.

STORAGE AND TRANSFORMATION

In addition to its other roles, the liver stores sugars, fats, and vitamins until they are needed. It stores glycogen, a complex carbohydrate that is converted to sugar for release into your bloodstream when your blood sugar levels fall. Glycogen is deposited in the liver when the level of sugar in the blood rises. The liver uses enzymes to transform small building blocks such as amino acids, sugars, and fatty acids into more complex helpful substances. The liver also inactivates some hormones, regulates the amount of testosterone and estrogen in the blood, and plays a major role in breaking down and building up cholesterol.

Your liver:

- *forms blood before birth*
- *produces quick energy when necessary*
- *manufactures new body proteins*
- *prevents shortages in fuel*
- *regulates transport of fat stores*
- *manufactures blood clotting components*

- *helps digestion*
- *destroys poisonous substances*
- *metabolizes alcohol*
- *regulates chemical and drug levels in the body*
- *cleanses the blood*
- *discharges waste products*
- *maintains hormone balance*
- *helps the body resist infection*
- *stores iron*

It might seem that the liver is extremely vulnerable because of its exposure to so many harmful substances, and it's certainly true that your liver is under major stress: Harsh, toxic substances such as alcoholic beverages, powerful medicines, and recreational drugs all place a heavy burden on this one vital organ.

However, nature has provided the liver with several ways to protect itself. First of all, unlike many other organs in the body, the liver can heal and replace its own damaged tissues—to a degree. And because it's built with so many units that are responsible for the same task, if a section of the liver is injured, other liver cells can take over and perform the same duties of the damaged cells indefinitely, until the liver can repair itself.

Despite this built-in protection, the liver is still affected by a variety of diseases. It is especially vulnerable to inflammatory diseases such as hepatitis, the medical term for an inflammation of the liver.

In the next chapter, you'll learn about the specific viruses that can cause hepatitis, including one of the most deadly of them all: hepatitis C, the new "mystery disease" labeled as a silent killer for its ability to exist undetected within your body for decades while quietly destroying liver cells.

CHAPTER 2

WHAT IS HEPATITIS C?

Hepatitis is a disease as old as the Greek and Roman hills. Hippocrates was the first to note the occurrence of jaundice epidemics—the telltale yellowing of the skin that heralds the fact that the liver can no longer properly cleanse the blood.

In fact, hepatitis is not really a single disease, but a term that means *inflammation of the liver.* Because the liver plays a central role in human metabolism, just about any virus is capable of affecting it. However, there are a number of viruses that seem expressly intent on infecting and damaging liver cells in particular—the so-called hepatitis virus that scientists have given separate initials: hepatitis viruses A, B, C, D, E, and G.

While they are all called hepatitis viruses, each of these alphabetical microbes belongs to a separate virus family. Hepatitis B and C viruses are the most deadly, but there is now a vaccine to protect against hepatitis B. At present, there is neither vaccine nor effective treatment for hepatitis C.

While most of us have only recently heard of hepatitis C, in fact the collective condition known as hepatitis has sickened many people over the centuries and found many victims on the world's battlefields. During the Civil War alone, at least 70,000 soldiers fell under the scourge of infectious hepatitis. Eventually, scientists noticed that hepatitis appeared to be linked to a portion of patients who had been given blood, suspecting that the cause must be transmitted in the donated blood. By the beginning of World War II, doctors had identified two types of hepatitis and were able to differentiate between them based on how they were spread: *infectious hepatitis* was carried in contaminated food or water; *serum hepatitis* was transmitted via blood.

However, while the acute, infectious form of hepatitis had been recognized since 1885, the cause of that infection—the hepatitis B virus—was not identified until the 1960s, in the wake of a horrifying hepatitis epidemic at the Willowbrook State School for the Mentally Handicapped in Long Island, New York, where filthy living conditions sickened almost 100 percent of the patients. Eventually, doctors were able to isolate hepatitis A virus in 1973.

But this still left many cases that were not caused by either virus. Hepatitis patients who tested negative for hepatitis A or B viruses were said to be infected with a mysterious third virus, known as non-A, non-B hepatitis. It is now known that the majority of these patients with the mystery virus were in fact infected with hepatitis C virus (HCV), which was discovered in 1987. As tests for this virus have improved since 1989, more and more patients who have non-A, non-B hepatitis are now being correctly diagnosed.

Scientists believe that the HCV genotypes we recognize today were all derived from an original strain that developed about 100 to 120 years ago—a relatively recent infection compared to other human viruses. Although HCV has been classified into only several main types, in fact there are hundreds of different genetic identities; doctors believe that hepatitis C consists of a family of viruses with a variety of subtypes.

Some experts believe that HCV originated in the Far East because of the diversity and numbers of people infected in that part of the world. Strains found recently in Thailand suggest that the virus has been mutating for a long time in Asia. Because so many of the HCV patients in Japan are elderly, experts suspect that the blood supply was contaminated during the second World War or shortly afterward. There are similarities in the genotypes of older Japanese patients and those of older U.S. hemophiliacs. Moreover, military men in the Far East may have received local blood transfusions, then gone home and become blood donors, spreading the infection. It was at this time that the world's blood transfusion industry was becoming international in scope. Because HCV is so infectious, it only takes a small blood sample to contaminate large parts of the blood supply.

By the 1970s and 1980s more and more patients began showing up with non-A, non-B hepatitis. It was the Japanese who first noticed the rising rates of cirrhosis and liver cancer and believed that some pathogen might be the cause. At the same time, Western doctors began to realize that hemophiliacs were becoming infected with non-A, non-B hepatitis, but they couldn't find the cause in the nation's blood supplies.

Studies of patients with non-A, non-B hepatitis found an association between the disease and a recent history of blood transfusion, injected drug abuse, health care employment, sexual or household exposure to someone with hepatitis, multiple sex partners, or poor socioeconomic position. In 1989 scientists successfully identified the pathogen as hepatitis C.

Today, scientists have isolated six different and unrelated hepatitis viruses—termed A, B, C, D, E, and G. Four other viruses that are believed to cause hepatitis have been identified, but not much is known about them. While each of the following hepatitis viruses are caused by different things, they all produce liver inflammation. Hepatitis B and C are considered to be the most serious and affect the most people; both can become chronic (lasting longer than six months) and lead to serious liver damage such as cirrhosis and liver cancer. Infection with one form of the hepatitis viruses does not protect you against getting any or all of the others.

Hepatitis A Virus (HAV)   Formerly known as *infectious hepatitis,* HAV is the least dangerous of all viral forms of hepatitis. It is also the most easily prevented, since it is spread through contaminated water and food and is excreted in stools; there have been more than thirty U.S. outbreaks in the past fifteen years. The HAV resembles the polio virus and is a fairly simple structure with not more than a single strand of RNA genetic material in a twenty-sided shell that reproduces only in the liver. One of the "filth viruses," it usually appears wherever sanitation and personal hygiene are poor. Widespread epidemics are no longer common in the United States, but there may be isolated waves of infection at day-care centers, in polluted water, or in shellfish harvested from contaminated water. HAV can develop in as few as two weeks after exposure, but children don't usually have serious symptoms. While they are almost never jaundiced, they can transmit the infection to adults who do show the typical yellow eyes and skin, nausea and vomiting, and dark urine. In addition, adults who travel to places where hepatitis A is widespread can suffer more serious problems.

The new hepatitis A vaccine (Havrix) is very effective and is typically given in two doses six months apart. Travelers should have the first dose administered at least three weeks before departure to an area where hepatitis A is endemic, and also may want to receive standard gamma globulin to ensure protection. Protection from the vaccine lasts for at least three years. At this time, the need for booster doses is not clear, although scientists suspect that (like hepatitis B) they would be unnecessary.

Hepatitis B Virus (HBV)   A much more complex and serious virus than HAV, HBV was distinguished clinically from infectious hepatitis (hepatitis A) in the 1930s. Like hepatitis C, HBV is known as a "quiet killer;" it can be transmitted in contaminated blood or blood products, or via a tiny cut or abrasion. It also can be transmitted in semen, which places it on the list of venereal diseases. Finally, hepatitis B can be transmitted during toothbrushing, ear piercing, tattooing, dental work, or childbirth. Because the virus is extremely stable, it can remain on contaminated needles, surgical tools, and even thorns or sharp stones. It may take as long as six months to produce symptoms, versus just six weeks for hepatitis A. Before routine testing of the U.S. blood supply in 1990, hepatitis B killed thousands of people every year; today, millions of people around the world are still chronically infected and capable of passing on the infection. In Asia and Africa, hepatitis B is commonly passed from mother to child during birth or breast feeding. Like hepatitis C, the germ can eventually lead to liver cancer. All blood, organ, and tissue donations in developed countries are now tested for HBV, and risk of transmission in these areas is extremely low. A vaccine was licensed in 1982.

Hepatitis C Virus (HCV) Today, four million Americans are infected with HCV, and up to 30,000 new cases are reported each year. At the moment, the disease is responsible for about 8,000 to 10,000 deaths each year—and without effective treatment, that number is expected to triple in the next ten to twenty years. Hepatitis C is now the leading cause of liver transplantation in the United States. Three out of every four people who become infected with hepatitis C will be infected for life, and up to half of those will go on to develop cirrhosis (scarring of the liver).

Hepatitis D Virus (delta hepatitis) This virus can only thrive in cells also infected with hepatitis B since it needs the B virus's coating material to survive.

Hepatitis E Virus Believed to be transmitted through the feces of an infected person or by eating food contaminated by feces (especially raw shellfish), rather like hepatitis A, this type can occur in epidemics and is sometimes called *non-A, non-B, non-C hepatitis.* It is newly recognized as the cause of major epidemics in Asia, Africa, and Mexico. While the normal course of infection appears to be an acute but relatively harmless illness, infection during pregnancy carries a 15 to 30 percent mortality rate. Recombinant vaccines for this type of hepatitis virus are currently being prepared.

Hepatitis G Virus (HGV) Although transmitted through infected blood products, HGV does not appear to cause serious liver damage, according to government research reports in the *New England Journal of Medicine.* The virus, first identified in 1995, appears to be common in the United States. Patients infected with HGV either develop no symptoms or recover quickly after a mild illness. In a patient with both HGV and HCV infections, the hepatitis G infection does not appear to worsen severity of symptoms. On the other hand, scientists caution that the new virus might still be harmful in other, unknown ways and recommend further study.

Other Possible Viruses The GBV-C virus is associated with acute and chronic forms of hepatitis in humans and was originally isolated from a surgeon who died in 1994. Scant data on this virus now available suggest that it can lead to a fulminant form of hepatitis. Other reports suggest there are still other hepatitis viruses, such as HFV. Some scientists suspect this may suggest the existence of still other hepatitis viruses as yet undescribed.

WHAT IS THE HEPATITIS C VIRUS?

Hepatitis C is a single-stranded RNA virus. Because there are many closely related genetic forms of the virus (called *genotypes*), scientists suspect the virus has the ability to escape detection by the body's immune system, which leads to a high rate of chronic infection. This genetic diversity may explain why there are such wide differences in the way patients experience symptoms and respond to treatment.

Researchers have divided the hepatitis C virus into at least six major groups, called types or genotypes, designated 1 through 6. Each genotype contains up to three subtypes (labeled 1a, 1b, 1c, 2a, 2b, and so on). Some genotypes of hepatitis C appear to be restricted to certain areas of the globe, while others are found all over the world. Types 1a and 1b account for more than 60 percent of all infections in North America; types 2a and 2b and types 3 and 4 account for the rest. Except in Quebec, type 5 is rarely found in North America, but is common in South Africa. Type 4 is commonly found in central Africa and the Middle East, but is rare in Europe. Type 6 is most common in Hong Kong.

In one U.S. study, 58 percent of patients had genotype 1a, 21 percent had 1b, 2 percent had 2a, 13 percent had 2b, 5 percent had 3a, and 1 percent had 4a. There was no association between the type of genotype and the way the person had acquired the infection, but the study did find that those with genotypes 1a and 1b had the most severe hepatitis.

Most experts believe that infection with type 1b leads to the most aggressive disease, responds less well to interferon, and recurs more quickly after liver transplant. People with type 1b infection tend to be older and have acquired their infection from a transfusion instead of injected drug abuse.

As much as experts understand about the different species of hepatitis C, genotyping this virus is still in the experimental stages. Genotype testing is not widely available; a person can be tested only at certain research institutions (such as Stanford University). Moreover, while genotyping may be useful in determining who responds better to interferon, experts say it should not be used to determine who is suitable for treatment and who is not.

In addition to the genotype of hepatitis C, a person may also have in his liver and bloodstream a number of variant genomes of the same genotype (called *quasispecies*) or swarms of closely related but different viruses that originate from the same infecting virus. Quasispecies may become more diverse over time and may contribute to interferon resistance.

More extensive genetic analysis of hepatitis C virus has revealed that dividing the different species into types, subtypes, and such is somewhat artificial. Instead, the virus probably exists as a continuum of genetic diversity, according to Robert H. Purcell, M.D., head of the hepatitis section at the laboratory of infectious diseases, National Institute of Allergy and Infectious Diseases (NIAID).

Because the virus is so genetically diverse, it can evade your body's immune surveillance. This evasion leads to a high rate of chronic infections and lack of immunity to reinfection in people who are exposed more than once.

Recently, researchers have for the first time been able to isolate an infectious clone of the hepatitis C virus, proving that the virus alone can cause disease. This major development will profoundly influence the field of research, helping scientists better understand the factors that determine whether the virus is cleared from the body or produces a chronic infection, according to Anthony S. Fauci, M.D., director of NIAID. Since the virus was first discovered in 1989, scientists have detected HCV genetic sequences and antibodies in patients with classic non-A, non-B hepatitis and were able to screen the nation's blood supply for hepatitis C. But until now, scientists were not able to grow the virus efficiently in tissue culture or purify it using other lab procedures. These are all necessary steps in the process of verifying that a suspected infectious agent does in fact cause disease. This is why there have been questions about whether the HCV genetic sequences found in patients were really what caused the disease.

When you come in contact with the virus, hepatitis C first enters your bloodstream and then passes through your liver, where it enters liver cells and begins to reproduce. Your body's immune system tries to fight off this foreign invader, causing the liver to become inflamed.

Far less deadly than human immunodeficiency virus (HIV) but quite persistent, HCV can be detected in blood within one to three weeks after infection. Within an average of fifty days, most patients develop liver cell injury but probably won't know that a deadly fight is going on inside their bodies between their immune systems and the virus. While a few victims become sick with flu-like symptoms for a few weeks after initial exposure, most people have no symptoms at all.

Still, antibodies to HCV produced by the immune system usually can be detected in up to 70 percent of patients who experience symptoms and in about 90 percent of patients three months after infection. The antibody takes six weeks to six months after a person is infected to appear in the blood; in 10 percent of patients, it may take as long as a year before the test can detect the antibody. Patients are infectious as long as the virus remains in the blood—this can be for years. Still, hepatitis C is much more difficult to transmit in person-to-person contact than other infectious diseases such as chronic hepatitis B because the levels of circulating virus are much lower. On the other hand, it is fairly easy to transmit hepatitis C by injection (either blood transfusion or drug abuse).

A person's chance of becoming a carrier if infected by hepatitis C is at least 60 percent. Recent studies have shown that most carriers after twenty years had not developed liver disease, however, and did not die any sooner than noninfected people. That is, while these carriers have chronic infection, the virus is not damaging their livers. More severe liver disease is associated with hepatitis C patients who also are elderly or who have alcoholism, hepatitis B, or HIV infection.

WHO GETS HCV?

Hemophiliacs and drug abusers are at highest risk but anyone can acquire this virus; many people who have the virus don't know how they acquired it. From 20 to 40 percent of patients in inner-city hospitals have hepatitis C, as do 80 percent of drug users. The infection is more common in minority groups (3.2 percent of African Americans and 2.1 percent of Mexican Americans) than in non-Hispanic whites (1.5 percent). Homosexual transmission of hepatitis C is relatively uncommon; French investigators estimate the prevalence of infection to be about 5.3 percent among homosexual men with chronic hepatitis, but the more partners the higher the risk in this group.

You are at risk for hepatitis C if you have:

- *injected drugs*
- *had a job that exposed you to human blood*
- *had hemodialysis*
- *received a blood transfusion before 1992*
- *received blood products before 1992*
- *received a blood transfusion or blood products overseas*

You *may* be at risk for hepatitis C if you have:

- *had multiple sex partners*
- *lived with a person who has hepatitis C*

Also, contaminated batches of Gammagard and Polygam (drugs used in IV immunoglobulin therapy) may have caused thousands of infections across the United States (mostly children). Gammagard is primarily used to boost a patient's immune system. If you have received immunoglobulin therapy with Gammagard, you should contact your doctor immediately to have liver function tests.

CHRONIC INFECTION

Most patients who are infected with hepatitis C first experience symptoms similar to the flu, except that this illness doesn't completely go away. But for many others, the onset of hepatitis C is very gradual. Infants and young children may not have any symptoms at all.

Hepatitis C is considered to be *chronic* if it lasts for more than six months.

Only about 15 percent of people who become infected with HCV are able to fight off the virus completely and recover. Those who do rarely have any symptoms of the disease. The remaining 85 percent fail to clear the virus within six months and develop long-term (chronic) infection. During the first twenty years after infection, with only occasional exceptions, the disease causes few problems.

If cirrhosis does develop during this period, the patient is more likely to go on to develop fatal liver problems. The proportion of people whose disease remains completely stable isn't yet known, but it may well be a majority. Antibodies to HCV can be found in almost all patients with chronic hepatitis.

Most people with chronic hepatitis C don't have any symptoms or illness when they are first infected, and they often feel perfectly healthy for many years, despite the presence of the infection. The 15 percent of patients with chronic hepatitis who recover without treatment will have the virus disappear from the blood and have a return of normal liver enzymes. In most cases, chronic hepatitis C proceeds slowly, although this rate of progression varies a great deal from one person to the next. Symptoms first appear in many patients with chronic HCV when they begin to develop advanced liver disease. (See Chapter 3 for details about symptoms.)

However, if you have chronic hepatitis C infection, it's important for you to understand that although your infection will last for decades, in the majority of cases chronic HCV does not end in debilitating disease or early death. It is still difficult, however, to predict which patients will do well and which won't. Scientists don't understand why some people recover from HCV and others go on to develop complications. It does appear that the older the patient is when infected, the faster the disease progresses. Other possible influences include race and gender.

COMPLICATIONS

Unfortunately, in a few cases hepatitis C infection can lead to serious liver disease. Chronic long-term inflammation of the liver can lead to scarring as the liver attempts to protect itself from the inflammation. Doctors call this process *cirrhosis,* and chronic infection with hepatitis C is now recognized as one of the most common causes of cirrhosis. Of course, not everyone with chronic hepatitis C—even after many years—will develop cirrhosis, and there is a great variation in the rate at which cirrhosis develops. Some people may have cirrhosis within five years of becoming infected with hepatitis C, but others won't have cirrhosis even fifty or sixty years later. At least 20 percent of patients with chronic HCV will develop cirrhosis over a twenty- to thirty-year period. Occasionally, cirrhosis and end-stage liver disease occur rapidly, especially among those who abuse alcohol.

Many patients with cirrhosis will still remain healthy for many years, but a few can develop liver cancer as a complication of cirrhosis. This increased risk of liver cancer occurs among people with cirrhosis from all causes, not just hepatitis C. The actual risk of developing liver cancer at any point after becoming infected with the hepatitis C virus is not known, but it may be as high as a 25 percent increased risk, with a death rate between 5 and 10 percent. On the other hand, people with hepatitis C who don't have cirrhosis have no higher risk of liver cancer than those without the infection.

Whether or not a person develops complications appears to have something to do with cultural or environmental influences that are as yet not understood. Complications may be related to infection with other viruses, exposure to environmental pollutants, cigarette smoking, or chronic alcoholism. Complications may also be related to the amount of virus in the body, the genotype, and other viral species. In fact, infection with both hepatitis B and C has been reported to increase the severity of chronic hepatitis C and the likelihood of developing liver cancer. Among hemophiliacs, infection with both HCV and HIV boosts the HCV levels and leads to a worsening of the course of the disease. Chronic alcoholism clearly worsens the progression of hepatitis C, either because it boosts the reproduction of the virus or because it also damages the liver.

PREGNANCY AND HEPATITIS C

Pregnancy has very little effect on a normal liver; while there are no significant changes in liver function, certain markers of liver function will change slightly during a normal pregnancy. (For example, there may be lower levels of protein albumin because of the dilution of your blood.) In addition, the blood levels of alkaline phosphatase, which is usually taken to be an indicator of liver disease, may increase in a normal pregnancy because the placenta will produce this marker. This small change does not indicate liver disease.

Doctors now recommend that all pregnant women be tested during the last two or three months of pregnancy for the presence of the hepatitis B virus, but not the hepatitis C virus. This is because babies born to women who carry the hepatitis B virus are at considerable risk of developing hepatitis B right after delivery. If doctors know about the mother's condition, they can vaccinate the baby right after birth and give the child a special gamma glob-ulin preparation for immediate protection. These measures can prevent most cases of hepatitis B in babies whose mothers are infected.

On the other hand, babies born to women with hepatitis C are very unlikely to contract the disease themselves. However, it is remotely possible that transmission of the virus can occur. Unfortu-nately, there is no way at present to prevent this. For this reason, preg-nant women are not tested for the hepatitis C virus.

If you do have hepatitis C, you can still become pregnant if your liver is not seriously damaged. If you have had a liver transplant, you can still get pregnant; there have been women with hepatitis C who have had healthy children after undergoing successful liver transplants.

While it is not known if the hepatitis C virus can be transmitted in breast milk, it seems to be a low risk. A nursing mother may take interferon to treat her hepatitis C infection. However, it is not known if the drug will have any effect on the nursing baby. Because of this, doctors will usually try to give you interferon either before you get pregnant or after you have finished nursing.

If your liver is not so healthy—that is, if you have developed cirrhosis—it is still possible to become pregnant, although you will have markedly decreased fertility. If you do become pregnant, you may give birth to a healthy baby, but you may experience complications of liver failure during pregnancy. If so, your baby is at higher risk of premature delivery, spontaneous abortion, miscarriage, and stillbirth. Those children who are born, however, are usually healthy. For most people, hepatitis C will not interfere with their lifestyle or employment. Although fatigue is common in viral hepatitis, it is hard to blame it on the disease itself. In addition, fatigue rarely improves during interferon therapy, even if patients respond well to therapy. Neither prolonged bed rest nor strenuous exercise will affect the course of the disease. Patients should maintain their normal level of activity.

How It Is Transmitted

Hepatitis C is a blood-borne virus transmitted primarily through blood contamination. It is known to have survived in dried blood for longer periods than many other viruses (such as HIV)—possibly as long as three months. Since experts have not determined its survival period, however, no safe limit has been defined. Because HCV is so small and often lives in blood cells, it can survive for as long as those blood cells remain intact. The virus exists primarily in the liver and in various components of blood, but not in most other parts of the body.

While nobody can explain the source of up to half of all known cases of infection, the best known link to the disease is through blood contamination and shared needles. Those who received blood transfusions before 1992 are at risk, since blood was not screened for HCV at all before 1990, and the screening process was not as effective between 1990 and 1992 as it is today. The 1990 screening test was not accurate enough to diagnose hepatitis C.

It's also possible to transmit the disease via shared tools that come in contact with blood, such as manicure scissors, toothbrushes, or razors.

The following people are considered high-risk individuals and are potential candidates for hepatitis C screening:

- *anyone with hepatitis signs or symptoms*
- *anyone with unexplainably high liver enzymes*
- *intravenous drug users (past or present)*
- *anyone with a needle-stick injury*
- *anyone who is sexually active with multiple partners*
- *hemodialysis patients*
- *health care workers with exposure to blood or blood products*
- *anyone who has had a transfusion or received blood products*
- *transplant recipients*
- *anyone with a tattoo*
- *institutionalized people (including prisoners)*
- *infants of infected mothers*
- *police, firefighters, or anyone exposed to blood products at work*

As far as medical researchers can determine, the virus is *not* spread by:

- *the air, food, or water*
- *kissing*

- *sneezing or coughing*
- *using the same bathroom as an infected person*
- *eating food prepared by an infected person*
- *swimming in the same pool with an infected person*
- *holding an infected child*

BLOOD TRANSFUSIONS, OPERATIONS, AND INFECTED BLOOD PRODUCTS

Anyone who received a blood transfusion or blood products before 1992 is considered to be at high risk, since the primary route for transmission of HCV in the past was via contaminated blood in transfusions or blood products. In August 1997 U.S. government advisers recommended that anyone who had a blood transfusion before 1992 should be tested for hepatitis C. In addition, the panel recommended that blood banks across the nation check their records for any donors who have tested positive for hepatitis C since 1992, and then trace records of any recipients of blood from those donors back to 1987. Those recipients who received tainted blood must be notified by a letter that they should be tested.

One reason why this is particularly important is that recent research suggests hepatitis C patients who are infected through contaminated blood are especially vulnerable to liver failure.

About 290,000 Americans got hepatitis C from transfusions before the first tests for the virus were created in 1990. But because that first test needed improvements, it wasn't until mid-1992 that blood banks had truly effective screening tests for hepatitis C. Since 1992, however, the rate of new cases appears to be declining from its 1989 peak. The risk of transfusion-related hepatitis today is believed to range between 1 in 10,000 units to 1 in 100,000 units, according to the National Institutes of Health (NIH).

Still, nearly all hemophiliacs who were born before 1986 have hepatitis C.

Drug Use

Today, the most common way to transmit hepatitis C is through injected drugs. It's important to remember that not everybody who contracted hepatitis C in this way is—or was—a heavy drug user or shared needles for injection. Simply sharing a container with a liquid drug preparation that several people use together to fill syringes is enough blood-to-blood contact to spread hepatitis C. Since many drug abusers are believed to have been infected in the 1960s, many people who used drugs then but haven't touched a needle since may be infected.

In general, the group of people infected via drug abuse paraphernalia tend to be younger than those infected via transfusions. Moreover, those who contracted the disease through occasional IV drug abuse are likely to have a better prognosis and lower amount of virus in the blood. Long-term drug abusers are more likely to be infected with multiple strains of virus, meaning they may be more difficult to treat. These patients also tend to be generally less healthy and may also be alcoholic, which influences the course of their hepatitis.

Tattooing and Body Piercing

Since HCV is spread by contaminated blood, it is possible to transmit the virus via contaminated needles used in body piercing or tattooing. If you get a tattoo or you plan on having your body pierced, make sure the equipment is either previously unused, sterilized at high temperatures, or bathed in special sterilizing fluids.

Some experts estimate that between 1 and 2 percent of all cases of hepatitis C were caused by this method of transmission.

Acupuncture and Vaccination

Some hepatitis C cases in developing countries are related to poorly sterilized acupuncture or vaccination needles, as well as by practices that require skin piercing or other types of folk medicine. Invasive medical procedures conducted under less-than-sterile conditions may also lead to the transmission of HCV.

In the developed countries, acupuncture needles are vigorously sterilized before reuse or are used only once and discarded.

HOUSEHOLD CONTACT

Because the virus is hard to kill and can exist in almost-invisible amounts of blood, it is possible to spread HCV through sharing or touching personal care products that contain blood, such as razors, tweezers, nail clippers, scissors, toothbrushes, water pics, tampons, or sanitary napkins. Some estimates suggest that up to 2 percent of all hepatitis C cases are spread this way. The chance of transmission rises over time; therefore, those sharing a toothbrush for many years have a higher risk of transmitting the virus.

So far, there has not been any evidence of HCV transmission among nonsexual partners within households in which a patient is living.

One new study found that barbers who rely on nondisposable, nonsterilized blades to shave their customers run the risk of contracting hepatitis C—and their customers may face the same threat. In a French study of Sicilian barbers who shaved with the same instruments they used on their customers, 38 percent had antibodies to HCV. In comparison, a control group of people being screened as blood donors showed no evidence of blood infection. In Italy, up to 1.5 percent of the general population carries hepatitis C.

HEMODIALYSIS

Unfortunately, hepatitis C is fairly commonly found in hemodialysis units, according to some studies. In one Tufts University study, the rate of infection among dialysis patients without a history of blood transfusion was 16 percent, a rate much higher than that found in the general population.

HEALTH CARE WORKERS

It's possible to be exposed to HCV in any job where you may come in contact with blood. These higher-risk workers include nurses, phlebotomists, emergency medical workers, police and firemen, and so on.

The risk of infection after a needle-stick injury with contaminated blood may be as high as 10 percent. However, in recent studies only 3 out of 174 health care workers stuck by needles from infected patients went on to test positive for HCV. There has been evidence that infected surgeons have transmitted hepatitis C to their patients, although it is not known if certain types of surgery pose a higher risk than other types. In Britain and the United States, infected surgeons and obstetricians are allowed to continue unrestricted practice unless they have transmitted infection to a patient.

MOTHER-CHILD

Since the risk of maternal transmission is low, pregnant women are not routinely screened for hepatitis C infection. While mother-to-infant transmission of hepatitis C has occurred, it seems that it is not very easy, according to the National Institutes of Health. Weighing the often-conflicting reports about mother-infant transmission, the Centers for Disease Control estimates the likelihood is probably between 5 and 6 percent, although if the mother is also HIV positive the risk of passing on HCV as well is much higher. The risk is also higher if the mother has a higher concentration of virus in her blood. Even in Japan, where a much more severe version of HCV is common, only 6 percent of babies born to infected mothers contracted the disease.

Most babies born to infected mothers have a temporary accumulation of antibodies to the hepatitis C virus from their mothers. Studies of up to two years after birth found that infants of infected mothers did not contract the disease. However, experts caution that so far researchers have studied only a small number of infants; there may be a delayed onset that has not yet appeared. While it is true that the risk is low, there is still a possibility that an infant could be infected. Chronic infection usually develops in children who contract hepatitis C before or shortly after birth.

Hepatitis C has been found in breast milk, but there have been no reports of infection as a result of breastfeeding, and doctors don't prohibit infected mothers from breastfeeding.

INSECTS

It is considered to be highly unlikely that the hepatitis C virus can be carried by mosquitoes, since the amount of virus in the body is considered to be too low to be picked up by biting insects. Research exploring whether the virus can replicate in mosquito cells has failed to prove that it does.

SALIVA

The virus is not normally present in saliva, but transmission in saliva containing blood or by a human bite, has been reported. There are conflicting research reports about whether or not the virus may occasionally be found in either saliva or tear fluid.

OXYGEN MASKS

According to reports from Australia, some patients appear to have contracted hepatitis C from tiny traces of blood in the filters of anesthesia masks.

UNKNOWN SOURCES

In about 40 percent of cases, people who have been diagnosed with hepatitis C infection can't recall any risk factors and don't know how they acquired the infection. Some of these people probably have used injected drugs, received injections as a child with nondisposable needles, had blood transfusions they didn't know about during surgery, or were exposed to another person's blood in some way they don't recall. Some experts believe that a fair portion of these cases may be caused by things such as tattooing, body piercing, and even manicures. However, as of 1995, experts admit they may not have identified all the ways it's possible to transmit this virus.

SEXUAL INTERCOURSE

It is theoretically possible to transmit hepatitis C through unprotected sex, although research studies have reached different conclusions on this risk. Estimates suggest the rate may be up to 2.5 percent for prolonged sexual exposure. (Those with frequent sexual partners, such as prostitutes, promiscuous homosexual men, and those attending clinics for sexually transmitted diseases, may have a 20 percent risk.)

The hepatitis C virus is not present in most body secretions, including semen, urine, and saliva, unless they contain blood particles. Doctors believe this method of transmitting the virus is not very efficient and that it doesn't occur very often. However, it is true that the overall hepatitis C virus infection rate is higher in sexually promiscuous groups. Some estimates suggest that one case in twenty can be traced to infection via sexual intercourse with a virus carrier, exposure to contaminated saliva, or other forms of intimate contact with an infected person.

While doctors recommend that regular sexual partners of HCV patients be tested, the risk of transmission is believed to be low. Experts say there is no logical reason for couples in long-standing monogamous relationships to use barrier sexual methods once a diagnosis has been given. However, young people who are sexually active with a variety of partners should use condoms for all casual sexual contact.

Still, the decision about whether or not to use safe sex barrier methods because of infection is a controversial area. Some doctors advise patients there is no risk of transmitting HCV through sex, while others recommend that you should always use a barrier method, such as a condom. Recent research does support the fact that transmission risk is possible.

Since hepatitis C has been found in menstrual blood, and because it is theoretically possible to infect your partner during sex if you are menstruating, women with HCV should avoid sex during menstruation until several days after the period ends. There is also the possibility that the virus may be transmitted via the genital herpes virus present in genital lesions of infected partners.

Prognosis

As serious as it can be, hepatitis C does not carry an automatic death sentence: it can be a benign disorder with no symptoms, or it can lead to a chronic problem linked to progressive liver disease, cirrhosis, and liver cancer.

About 85 percent of HCV infected people will clear the virus from their blood by six months, but the infection will persist in the liver and white cells. Eventually, they will develop chronic hepatitis with a persistent, but often intermittent, level of virus in the blood. The majority of patients with chronic infection will have abnormal ALT levels (a type of liver function test) that can fluctuate. About one-third of HCV patients will have normal ALT levels. This insidious disease may progress at a slow rate, with no symptoms or physical signs in most people, during the first twenty years after infection. A small portion of these patients (less than 20 percent) develop nonspecific symptoms, including fatigue and malaise. Many patients notice symptoms first when they begin to develop advanced liver disease.

The rate of progression is variable. Chronic infection leads to cirrhosis in at least 20 percent of patients within twenty years after onset of infection, although cirrhosis may sometimes develop quickly—especially if the patient drinks alcohol. After thirty years, about 1 to 5 percent of patients with chronic HCV will develop liver cancer. The ultimate prognosis for patients with the chronic form of the disease is not easy to predict since it seems to be affected by a variety of factors. Indeed, decades-long studies have found that those who received blood transfusions showed no difference in overall death rates between those who had HCV and those who were not infected with the virus.

CHAPTER 3

SYMPTOMS: HOW DO YOU KNOW IF YOU HAVE HEPATITIS C?

Sharon, 35, had no idea she had hepatitis C when she went to her doctor to find out more about the results of her blood screening. She had recently undergone an extensive batch of blood tests required by her insurance company when she wanted to apply for life insurance, and she had been denied.

Sharon had had a blood transfusion when she had started hemorrhaging after a cesarean section some years before, prior to the nation's blood supply screening for hepatitis C. The infection had slipped through—and infected Sharon.

Most people with hepatitis C don't know that anything is wrong with them when they first contract the disease. In the beginning, less than 5 percent show the classic symptoms of an acute attack and up to half of those infected may never experience any symptoms. The overall picture may differ markedly from one person to the next. You

Serious Complications

In more severe cases of chronic hepatitis C infection, patients may develop a variety of symptoms that are related to a poorly functioning liver (see Chapter 6). These include:

- swelling of abdomen and feet

- jaundice (yellow discoloration of eyes and skin)

- bruising more easily than normal

- intermittent confusion, disorientation, or inability to carry out mental tasks

Because the disease can silently destroy the liver for many years before symptoms occur, experts recommend that those who suspect they may have been exposed to the disease be tested.

may become infected and yet remain fairly healthy for decades, while your neighbor could contract the same virus and develop serious problems in just a few years. It does seem that people who become infected later in life get sick more quickly, although the progression rate also differs from one person to the next.

In those who do have symptoms, intermittent flare-ups tend to occur in cycles. For a while they may feel fine, and then they may go through days or weeks when they feel lousy. Some patients believe their condition improves in the spring and then worsens as September approaches, reaching its nadir in November or December.

Still, it's *not* true that hepatitis never causes any symptoms at all. Much is still not known about the hepatitis C virus, and many doctors who don't regularly treat the illness may not be familiar with the research describing its various symptoms. Some symptoms may be slight, or come and go. Many mimic other mild diseases and may be dismissed as just "some virus that's going around."

Within six to twelve weeks after infection, about a quarter to a half of patients who are infected with the hepatitis C virus report sudden flu-like symptoms that are very similar to mononucleosis— low fever, fatigue, nausea and vomiting, stomach pain, muscular aches, and loss of appetite. These symptoms of hepatitis C are indistinguishable from other types of acute viral hepatitis. About 10 percent become jaundiced, with yellowing of skin and eyes. Symptoms may appear from two weeks to six months after exposure, but usually occur within two months. Generally, these symptoms then eventually fade away. Other patients, however, notice the more gradual appearance of symptoms over a long period of time.

The rate at which infected patients go on to develop symptoms and the seriousness of these symptoms vary profoundly from one person to the next. Interestingly, the presence of symptoms in many people has nothing to do with how far along the illness has progressed. Someone with a mild infection may have many of the symptoms, while another person with a much more advanced case may not have any symptoms at all. Some people develop serious problems within five years, while others have no obvious liver symptoms for twenty years or more. Experts do believe that the older you are when first infected, the more serious the course of the disease.

If you have hepatitis C, within two weeks to six months after infection you may have:

- *appetite loss*
- *extreme fatigue*
- *nausea and vomiting*
- *stomach pain*
- *yellowing of skin and eyes (jaundice)*

Symptoms usually go away within two months. Half of those with symptoms go on to develop chronic liver disease (cirrhosis and cancer). But others who are infected have no symptoms at all and can infect others without being aware of their condition. Some of the most common symptoms include fatigue, itch, pain, appetite and weight loss, loss of libido, and "brain fog."

Children and Hepatitis C Symptoms

Infants and children with hepatitis C are less likely than adults to have symptoms of infection. For this reason, they are more likely to remain undiagnosed and are therefore more likely to spread the disease.

As far as researchers have been able to determine, children with chronic HCV still have normal growth patterns. Their long-term prognosis is presently believed to be about the same as that of an adult.

FATIGUE

The most common symptom hepatitis C patients experience is mild to debilitating fatigue (about 70 percent of patients have this problem). But the presence of fatigue alone hardly justifies a diagnosis of hepatitis C—fatigue can be attributed to many diseases. Even when it is a major complaint in someone known to have hepatitis C, the severity of the symptom is not usually directly related to the severity of the disease. Some people have disabling fatigue with very mild hepatitis C and no cirrhosis. Others have normal energy levels, while battling severe hepatitis C and cirrhosis.

Some people with hepatitis C believe they have chronic fatigue syndrome (known medically as myalgic encephalomyelitis). While isolated pockets of chronic fatigue syndrome have been found throughout the twentieth century, the syndrome became widely known during the 1980s, when it was identified by *Newsweek* magazine as "yuppie flu." Unlike hepatitis C (which has been strongly linked to drug addicts), people with chronic fatigue syndrome were believed to be primarily the upwardly mobile, hardworking young people who became ill due to stress and overwork. But researchers also strongly suspected an underlying viral cause, since many patients had abnormal ratios of helper T cells to killer cells—evidence that the immune system was responding to some type of infection. At various times, scientists suspected a link with herpes virus, cytomegalovirus, Epstein-Barr, and Coxsackie.

More recently, Australian researchers suggest that up to 40 percent of patients who were previously diagnosed with chronic fatigue syndrome in fact have hepatitis C. This doesn't necessarily mean there was a misdiagnosis; the two conditions could exist at the same time.

ITCH

Another common symptom is itchiness, often all over the body, without any skin rash. The cause of this itchiness is not well understood, although it is believed that the buildup of bilirubin in the skin may be related to the itching. It can be treated with antihistamines or cholestyramine (which binds to bile in the intestines).

PAIN

Many hepatitis C patients feel a variety of abdominal pains and discomfort, but unfortunately too often these pains are dismissed as having nothing to do with chronic liver disease. This is because abdominal organs are not responsive to many things that would normally elicit severe pain. The pain fibers in the large interior organs, such as the liver, are usually sensitive only to stretching or increased wall tensions—which is what happens as the liver becomes inflamed. About 20 percent of patients complain of pain over the liver area, in the right upper side of the abdomen just beneath the ribs. Some experts suspect this could be "referred pain" caused by inflammation and swelling of the covering of the liver. This pain also may occur in the right shoulder or to the back between the shoulder blades.

Pain that is caused by sensory nerves in the liver may cause a pain that is hard to describe—dull cramping or aching, appearing anywhere from the midline to the lower abdominal area. It may be accompanied by nausea and vomiting, sweating, pale skin, and restlessness during sleep.

Moreover, bacterial or viral infection of any organ in the abdominal area—including the liver—may cause abdominal pain.

APPETITE AND WEIGHT LOSS

About 15 percent of patients complain of loss of appetite, and 5 percent experience weight loss.

LOSS OF LIBIDO

If you have hepatitis C and you have lost interest in sex, you're not alone. Many patients have reported this problem, which may be related to depression or to interferon treatment. It's also likely related to stress, discomfort, and fatigue of the illness rather than any direct effect on hormonal levels.

BRAIN FOG

Some patients with hepatitis C have reported feeling as if their brains are stuffed with cotton wool. This "brain fog" is not the same thing as encephalopathy, a serious complication of hepatitis. Instead, it appears to be a milder form of concentration problem and occurs at all stages of the disease. Others complain of dizziness or blurry vision and dry eyes. Eye problems have also been related to interferon treatment.

There has been little research into the direct impact of HCV on the brain. However, the virus is known to infect certain blood cells and could be expected to reach the brain. Whether the virus causes damage once it gets there is not yet known, but patients do report many cognitive and mental problems.

In addition to the aforementioned most common symptoms, a wide variety of other symptoms have been reported by patients. Patients say that many of these symptoms seem to ebb and flow with the course of the disease:

- *abdominal bloating*
- *arthritis*
- *blood circulation problems*
- *blood sugar problems (type II diabetes)*
- *chest pains*
- *chills and fever*
- *depression*
- *diarrhea*
- *dizziness*
- *facial puffiness*
- *fatty food aversions*

- *female problems (irregular menses, severe PMS)*
- *fever (low grade)*
- *fluid retention*
- *headaches (frequent or continuous)*
- *indigestion*
- *irritable bowel syndrome*
- *joint pains or stiffness*
- *mental fatigue*
- *mood swings*
- *night sweats*
- *palpitations*
- *seasonal affective disorder*
- *sleep problems (not feeling rested)*
- *sore throat*
- *urination frequency (often during the night)*
- *urine discoloration (darkening)*
- *vivid dreams*

CHAPTER 4

DIAGNOSIS

*T*ori was a thirty-two-year-old writer living in Washington, D.C., when she got a letter in the mail following a visit to the Red Cross to donate blood. The people at the Red Cross were sorry, they told her, but her liver enzymes were elevated and they would have to reject her blood.

Liver enzymes? What in the world are they?

An active jogger and mother of two, she had no idea she was anything other than the healthy young woman she appeared to be. When she made an appointment with her family doctor, she learned that she was not healthy—somehow, she had contracted hepatitis C and even now it could possibly be silently destroying the cells deep within her liver. On hindsight, she *had* been tired lately, but she had attributed that to her busy schedule at work and at home.

Many people, like Tori, never suspect they have hepatitis C until they happen to run into a situation where their blood is tested. Perhaps

TABLE 4.1   Normal Value Ranges for Blood Tests
Relating to the Liver

A/G ratio	1.1–2.5
Albumin	g/dl 3.2–5.2
Alkaline phosphatase	u/l 39–117
ALT	u/l 0–31
AST	u/l 0–37
Bilirubin (total)	mg/dl 0.0–1.0
Gamma GT	u/l 7–33
Globulin (Calc)	g/dl 1.5–4.5
Iron	ug/dl 30-160
LDH	u/l 94-250
Protein (total)	g/dl 5.9–8.4

they're in one of the high-risk categories, they've tested positive during a blood donation screening, or they've had some abdominal pain.

If you think you might have some of the symptoms of hepatitis C, the first thing your doctor will do is conduct a physical exam. When your doctor taps the area of your abdomen above the liver, the resulting sound may indicate a change in the size and position of the liver. A normal liver is neither shrunken nor enlarged and is not tender to touch.

Other diseases will have to be ruled out. Your doctor will need to make sure you don't have hepatitis A or B, cytomegalovirus, Epstein-Barr, as well as nonviral liver problems such as fatty liver or substance abuse problems. If your doctor has any suspicion at all that you may have hepatitis C, the next step is to order tests. The diagnosis is most commonly made after the doctor detects an antibody to a portion of hepatitis C virus in your blood. The presence of this antibody indicates that you were exposed to the virus and that your immune system has produced an antibody to that virus. But because the test can show false positives (that is, indicate you have the infection when you really don't), your doctor will want to confirm the diagnosis by finding evidence that the virus is actually in your blood.

Before 1990, doctors could diagnose hepatitis C only by ruling out other possibilities (hence the former name for hepatitis C—non-A, non-B hepatitis). Detecting the hepatitis C virus has become much easier in the past several years, although it's still far from foolproof. To correctly diagnose hepatitis C, your doctor must confirm the presence of the virus infection and assess the severity of liver disease. Tests can also help determine whether or not you are likely to benefit from drug treatment, but there is no guarantee that you will respond.

In ordering some of these routine liver tests, the doctor doesn't usually have to request each one separately; they're done as a panel, called a *liver panel.* You should ask your doctor's staff to send you a copy of the results. These reports will list the results, as well as what the normal ranges (see Table 4.1) should be. You'll probably be able to get much more information by reading the tests yourself rather than relying on someone to read you the numbers over the phone.

HCV ANTIBODY DETECTION TESTS

The first diagnostic test your doctor will order is an antibody detection screening, called the *Enzyme Linked Immunosorbent Assay* (ELISA or EIA) that looks for antibodies to the hepatitis C virus in your blood—not the virus itself. These tests have improved a great deal in the short time they have been available. Current tests are accurate, with much lower false-negative and false-positive rates than in earlier years.

This test is crucial for early detection because acute hepatitis C infection is usually mild and tests of your liver function can sometimes be normal even though you have an HCV infection. However, while the antibody test will indicate if you have ever been infected, it can't tell the difference between an old and a new infection. It also can't distinguish between people who are infectious and those who have completely recovered. *Because it can take up to six months for antibodies to form in the blood, you should be retested six months after the first antibody test if you believe you might have been exposed to hepatitis C.* Only two-thirds of patients who go to their doctors with possible HCV infection can be diagnosed with blood tests for this reason.

If you were tested for HCV before 1995, you may want to confirm the results by having one of the more recent antibody tests or a polymerase chain reaction (PCR) test (see following section).

The *ELISA I* test introduced in 1991 looked for particular types of immune protein that corresponded to the presence of HCV antibodies. But this test tended to be unreliable, giving both false-positive and false-negative readings. It was replaced by *ELISA II* in 1993, which, due to its low cost and ease of administration, is often the initial test used to diagnose hepatitis C. *ELISA III,* even more sensitive than the last, is available, easy to perform, and inexpensive. Still, not all patients with active HCV infections are identified with the ELISA screening tests.

Supplemental tests for antibodies, called the *recombinant immunoblot assay (RIBA-3)* test, were developed to help with the false-positive readings. This test incorporates a search for two different sets of patterns in combination with checking for the presence of a control substance. The diagnosis of hepatitis C can be confirmed by this RIBA test, considered to be highly accurate—although still not 100 percent accurate. The RIBA detects antibodies to individual HCV antigens. Because the RIBA test costs more than the ELISA, this is usually used only to confirm the diagnosis.

The *Matrix test* is another antibody test that is considered to be highly accurate. It uses a technique called the *in vitro enzyme dot blot immunoassay.*

Because of the false-positive readings that occur with tests for HCV antibodies, supplementary tests for HCV infection should always be given to low-risk subjects who don't have any symptoms but who are found to have HCV antibodies in the blood—especially if liver function tests (discussed later in this chapter) are normal.

A small percentage (less than 10 percent) of patients may recover from acute HCV infection, but their anti-HCV test will remain positive. The anti-HCV test will remain positive for several years after a patient recovers from acute hepatitis C. Anyone who tests positive for the antibodies to HCV should undergo further testing to confirm the diagnosis. (See Table 4.2 for hepatitis C test results.)

VIRUS DETECTION AND ANALYSIS

If your doctor finds antibodies to the HCV virus, the next step is to look for the presence of the virus in the blood by finding nucleic acids associated with the virus (hepatitis C RNA) in the blood and body tissues. These tests tend to be more definitive than antibody tests, but they are also more expensive. In the *PCR* test—the most sensitive test available—a small section of the gene of the HCV RNA is amplified to detectable levels in the blood. The section is then pulled by an electric current through a gel made of clear seaweed compound. The size of the piece of gene is then compared with the known piece from hepatitis C. If they match, the test is positive. The test can be confirmed in several ways. The most precise way is to map the actual molecules in the piece of gene that is amplified and see if it matches the sequence of hepatitis C. This test can detect the virus within three days of infection.

Because recent studies suggest that the HCV RNA levels are relatively stable in untreated patients with chronic hepatitis C, the test can help identify the few patients infected with hepatitis C who have false-negative HCV antibody tests.

Unfortunately, the PCR test is not perfect. It may be more sensitive to some strains of hepatitis C virus than others, depending on the

TABLE 4.2   Hepatitis C Test Results

Test	Results	Interpretation	Recommendation
anti-HCV	positive	chronic hepatitis, chronic hepatitis C recovered, recent acute hepatitis C, or false-positive test	further evaluation
anti-HCV ALT supplemental test (RIBA-2)	positive normal positive	possible chronic HCV carrier, may have chronic hepatitis C	further evaluation
anti-HCV ALT supplemental test (RIBA-2)	positive elevated positive	presume chronic hepatitis C	further evaluation/ consider interferon therapy
anti-HCV ALT supplemental test (RIBA-2)	positive normal negative or indeterminate	presume false-positive anti-HCV or recovered	further evaluation by HCV-RNA PCR test if RIBA-2 negative or indeterminate
anti-HCV ALT supplemental test (RIBA-2)	positive elevated negative	presume false-positive anti-HCV, false-negative supplemental test unlikely	further evaluation for liver disease other than hepatitis C

Test	Results	Interpretation	Recommendation
ALT (no other symptoms)	elevated	possible fatty liver, chronic viral hepatitis, alcoholic liver disease, hemochromatosis, drug-induced liver injury, other liver diseases	further evaluation

genotype of the virus. But while it has its limitations, the PCR is probably the most useful single test for diagnosing hepatitis. It also can be used to determine whether hepatitis C treatment will be effective. But because of variability among testing labs, results must be interpreted cautiously. The National Institutes of Health HCV consensus panel has called for rigorous proficiency testing of clinical labs who perform this assay.

Understanding the results of these tests can be challenging. Having a negative PCR test doesn't necessarily mean that your infection has disappeared; the virus may just not be at high enough levels in the blood, or it may still be found in liver cells and in certain white blood cells. Some patients who appear to have cleared HCV from the blood in fact still have traces of the virus in their white blood cells. Moreover, it's possible to have antibodies to HCV in your blood but have no detectable HCV RNA. Conversely, some people who are infected with HCV RNA never develop antibodies.

If you do have a positive test result to any of the HCV screening tests and you have risk factors for hepatitis C or you have signs of liver disease, you probably have been infected with HCV. However, if you have no signs of liver disease and you don't engage in high-risk behavior, your hepatitis C "positive" could be a false-positive reading.

Contact your doctor to decide if your hepatitis C test result is accurate and whether you need more tests.

OTHER TESTS

While the preceding tests are the most common initial tests for hepatitis C, there are other options. The *b-DNA* for HCV (Quantiplex) is a less sensitive test for the virus in blood used as a quick way to assess infection levels and how much virus a person has. It estimates the viral load above a certain level; while the PCR can detect as little as 1,000 genomes, the b-DNA can detect levels over 350,000.

If you test negative, this doesn't mean you don't have the virus in your blood—you can be b-DNA-negative and PCR-positive. Some doctors believe that people who are b-DNA-negative have a good chance of responding to interferon treatment.

VIRAL LOAD

The PCR and other HCV RNA tests measure the *viral load,* or the amount of virus in your blood. The viral load can range from "not detected" to hundreds of millions. It's important to understand that the meaning of "not detected" or "negative" differs depending on the lab used. So if your doctor tells you that your viral load is negative, it may mean that you have no hepatitis C virus in your blood—or it may mean that you do have some virus, but the number of the viruses is lower than the detection limit of the lab.

To make things confusing, there are several ways to express the viral load. To compare different results, you have to know how to convert the numbers to a standard format—usually the plain number of how many viruses you have per milliliter—for example, 1.5 million/ml (or about 1,500,000/ml).

Sometimes the lab reports the amount of RNA material found by its weight. One picogram (pg) of genetic material corresponds to about

1 million virus equivalents, so if your lab results are given in picograms, multiply that result by 1 million and you have the number of viruses.

Alternatively, the viral load may be given as a plain number, such as 1.52 million, or 1,520,000, or 152000000. Sometimes, a lab abbreviates "millions" by the prefix "M"—so 1.52 Meq/ml means 1.52 Mega-equivalents/ml, or 1,520,000 equivalents/ml.

You might have a lab that reports large numbers in exponential form. To convert this to regular numbers, add as many zeroes to a 1 as the exponent says and multiply this with the number. If you see something like

Hep C RNA Quant 15.2 × 10 (exp) 5 equivalents/ml

you would translate this by adding five zeroes to the one, which gives you 100,000; multiply this by the number 15.2, which gives you 1,520,000 as the viral load.

GENOTYPES

The hepatitis C virus is a remarkably large family of viruses, with at least six distinct genotypes and many subtypes that have been identified throughout the world (see Chapter 2). You can find out which strain (or strains) of the HCV virus you have by taking a *genotype test.* Some genotypes are associated with more severe infections and poorer response to drug treatment, so it might seem that knowing your genotype could be important. However, the NIH consensus panel stresses that, at the moment, genotyping should be considered to be a research tool and not a part of diagnostic testing.

Still, it's possible to make some generalizations about genotype. The most serious hepatitis C genotype may be HCV 1b, because it is associated with more advanced liver disease. However, there is a wide difference in severity of liver disease associated with each genotype. Doctors don't fully understand the differences between the various genotypes and the implications of disease severity. Knowing your genotype could also be important if doctors can someday determine in detail which genotypes respond best to which types of interferon treatment.

At present, however, not everyone agrees that there is a link between the type of virus you have and how well you will respond to treatment. Some doctors believe that how much of the virus you have in your blood (viral load) is a more important factor in determining how well you respond to treatment.

In any case, the genotype tests fall into two categories: screening tests that detect mutations and tests that evaluate larger segments of HCV genes. Commonly used screening tests include *5′-RFLP analysis, coregene nested PCR,* and the *LIPA assay.* Confirmatory tests include *nucleotide sequencing* and *phylogenetic analysis of the E1 gene* or *NSSB gene.*

The tests are important in research, but because the tests are very expensive and difficult to administer, and because it's still not clear what the results may mean when it comes to treatment decisions, these tests aren't often performed in the doctor's office.

LIVER FUNCTION TESTS

Liver function tests are an important way of diagnosing liver disease, but they aren't always a good measure of how healthy your liver is if you have hepatitis C. Abnormal liver function tests suggest chronic disease, but there is no correlation between the level of the liver function tests and how severe your disease might be. Liver function tests, or a liver profile, are based on measuring the amounts of certain substances in the blood that are related to liver health:

- *ALT and AST (alanine aminotransferase and aspartate aminotransferase, two enzymes normally present in liver cells)*
- *bilirubin (a bile pigment extracted from the blood by the liver)*
- *albumin (a major protein found in the blood)*
- *alkaline phosphatase (a test that reveals biliary duct obstruction)*

- GGTP *(a test that pinpoints alkaline phosphatase levels)*
- *prothrombin time (a test of blood clotting efficiency)*
- *proteins (serum protein)—high levels are caused by liver inflammation (Al-antitrypsin, ceruloplasmin, transferrin, ferritin)*
- LDL *(cholesterol)*
- *globulin*

Different cells have different enzymes inside them depending on their function. As it happens, liver cells have a great deal of AST, ALT, and GGTP. When cells are damaged or die, these enzymes leak out into the blood. A higher level of these enzymes in your blood, then, indicates that something is wrong with your liver cells.

There are two general categories of liver enzymes. The first group are the indicators of liver cell damage: *alanine aminotransferase (ALT)* and *aspartate aminotransferase (AST)*. Tests of these two enzymes, then, can identify liver damage if the levels are very high. ALT is more specific for liver disease than AST, since AST is also found in more types of cells, including those of the heart, intestine, and muscle. Your AST, for example, will rise after you have a heart attack or a bruised kidney. An elevated liver enzyme level, a positive antibody test for HCV (anti-HCV), and negative tests for both hepatitis A and B infections probably mean that you have either active or chronic hepatitis C infection that is causing liver damage.

Very high ALT levels suggest viral hepatitis; moderate-to-high levels may indicate mononucleosis, chronic hepatitis, or early or improving acute viral hepatitis. Slight to moderate elevations (usually with higher increases in AST levels) appear in any condition that injures liver cells, such as active cirrhosis. Marginal elevations occur occasionally in heart attacks.

False (temporary) elevations of ALT may follow use of barbiturates, narcotics, methotrexate, chlorpromazine, aspirin, and any other drug that affects the liver.

The normal range for men is between 5 and 40 international units (iu) per liter (l), although some researchers say simply anything below 50 iu/l is normal. In women, the normal range is from 9 to 24 iu/l. (The normal range in infants is twice that of adults.)

However, many people with chronic hepatitis C infection—and who have hepatitis C RNA in their blood—have normal ALT blood levels. They usually don't have symptoms, and most have a mild liver disease with a good prognosis.

Still, these tests can only tell that there is some liver damage present—they can't determine how bad that damage is. A patient who has had elevated levels for only a few months is probably in better health than someone whose levels have been high for years—even if the first patient's levels are higher. And someone with cirrhosis may still have normal ALT and AST levels.

Remember that these tests are helpful, but they usually can't be interpreted without clinical information. They are probably most useful to track a particular problem, although they do tend to fluctuate in chronic hepatitis C. Even completely normal ALT readings do not ensure the virus has been eradicated. Because of this fluctuation, it's important to have the tests performed often in order to get a better understanding of the health of the liver.

The ALT is also sometimes known as the SGPT from its former name, serum glutamate pyruvate transaminase. AST may also be known as SGOT, from its former name serum glutamic-oxalacetic transaminase.

Other often-used tests of liver enzymes are measures of your *alkaline phosphatase* and *gamma-glutamyl transpeptidase (GGT)* that can indicate obstruction to the biliary system. The alkaline phosphatase test is used to uncover obstruction of the biliary system, which can be found in progressive liver disease. A high level of alkaline phosphatase suggests liver disease, such as hepatitis, cirrhosis, or liver cancer. (It's also possible to have high levels if you have gallstones or drug-induced hepatitis, or if you drink too much.) The normal range for this test is 35 to 130 iu/l.

Because alkaline phosphatase is also found in other organs (including bone, placenta, and intestines), your doctor may use a supplementary test—gamma-glutamyl transpeptidase (GGT)—to make sure the elevation of alkaline phosphatase is indeed coming from the liver or the biliary tract. The GGT is elevated in case of liver disorders, but is not elevated in diseases of bone, placenta, or intestine.

Although these tests are called "liver function tests," these tests don't really measure the liver function as such. To assess liver function, they must be corroborated with other tests, including those for albumin, bilirubin, and prothrombin time. Clinical factors also should be considered.

The next thing your doctor may want to do is to check your *bilirubin* levels. Bilirubin is the main bile pigment in humans which, when too high, causes the yellow discoloration of the skin and eyes called jaundice. Bilirubin is formed primarily from the breakdown of a substance in the red blood cells called *heme*. It is taken up from blood processed through the liver and then secreted into the bile by the liver. Healthy people have very little bilirubin in the blood (less than 1.2 mg/dL); higher levels may mean the red blood cells are being destroyed, that the bile flow from the liver is blocked, or that the liver is not functioning as well as it should. Levels above 3 mg/dL are usually noticeable as jaundice. Bilirubin levels in blood are usually considered to be a true test of liver function, since they reflect the liver's ability to take up, process, and secrete bilirubin into the bile.

A test that measures the *albumin* level of your blood can assess how effectively your liver forms protein. A problem in synthesizing protein could mean you have liver damage; chronic liver disease usually decreases the amount of albumin you produce. Normal albumin levels are between 35 to 50 g/l.

Still another measure of liver damage is the test of *prothrombin time (PT)*, which measures how efficiently your blood clots. When the liver is damaged, it may stop producing blood clotting factors. The PT is a useful test since there is a good correlation between abnormalities in coagulation (measured by PT) and the degree of liver dysfunction. PT is usually expressed in seconds and compared to a

What Do These Liver Tests Mean?

Alkaline phosphatase The level of alkaline phosphatase is elevated in various forms of hepatitis, cirrhosis, and liver cancer.

Bilirubin Levels are higher in liver disease, due to damaged liver.

GGT (glutamyl transpeptidase) These results will be elevated in liver disease.

LDH (lactic dehydrogenase) When very high, these results indicate cancer.

Liver enzymes Elevated levels indicate liver inflammation and nonspecific liver disease. In hepatitis C, the levels don't always correlate with severity of disease or symptoms.

Prothrombin time Increased prothrombin time indicates the malabsorption of vitamin K, which helps in clotting to prevent bleeding. Prothrombin time above five seconds indicates fulminant liver failure.

Proteins (serum proteins) These include AAT (al-antitrypsin), ceruloplasmin, transferrin, ferritin. Higher levels are caused by liver inflammation.

normal control patient's blood. Prothrombin time above five seconds indicates fulminant liver failure.

Interpretation of these tests (see sidebar for a summary) is a sophisticated process that your doctor will use together with your medical history, physical exam, and other tests—such as ultrasounds—to make a diagnosis.

ULTRASOUND SCANS

This nonintrusive method of testing the liver is a painless way of assessing liver health. While the test can't reveal detailed liver injuries, it's often possible to diagnose cirrhosis, which causes a distinctive lumpy, irregular surface. It also can reveal ascites (bloating) in the abdomen and detect liver or spleen enlargement. Ultrasound scans are usually done about once every year or two, depending on the level of your disease activity and whether you need to track down information about nonspecific symptoms.

In a liver ultrasound, you lie flat as the technician coats the skin over your liver area with a gel before sliding the microphone-shaped transducer over the skin. As this device moves along, inaudible high-frequency sound waves are passed into your body, where they bounce off the interface between tissues of different densities, such as fluid and air, or bone and muscle. The sound wave echoes are picked up by the transducer and transmitted by wires to an ultrasound machine that converts the electrical impulses into an image or picture of your liver that is displayed on the screen.

The procedure can be done on an outpatient basis. There is no pain and as far as scientists have been able to tell, no side effects.

LIVER BIOPSY

The best way of finding out the health of your liver is by having a *liver biopsy*, a minor surgical procedure that extracts a tiny sample of the liver with a needle so it can be examined under a microscope. The biopsy often helps doctors make a specific diagnosis when the cause of your liver disease isn't clear, and it can help determine the amount of liver damage you have. When you get your results, they are graded or "staged" as an indication of how much structural damage the liver has sustained.

Since the test is more sensitive and accurate than liver function tests, the biopsy can help confirm liver disease. It also provides information that can't be obtained by ALT tests alone. This is important, since it's possible to have normal ALT levels and still have significant liver disease. In fact, one study found that 70 percent of patients who tested positive for HCV antibodies in their blood but who had normal ALT levels did in fact have chronic hepatitis or cirrhosis, which was revealed when a liver biopsy was performed.

The need for biopsy may someday be eliminated as newer, more accurate liver function tests are developed. But as of today, it's still a useful tool in helping to understand the type of liver damage you may have.

THE PROCEDURE

The most common way to obtain a liver sample is by inserting a needle into the liver for a fraction of a second to remove a small piece of the liver. (This slight loss of tissue does not affect liver function.) Most of the time, doctors first order an ultrasound scan to determine the best, safest biopsy site and needle angle.

The skin and area under the skin are anesthetized and a needle is passed quickly into and out of the liver. General anesthesia is not used, but you can ask for IV sedation (such as Valium or Versed) to help you relax. It is important to be at least partially awake so you can hold your breath at certain points during the biopsy.

You'll be positioned flat on your back and given a local anesthetic. Your doctor will insert the thin needle between or below your ribs into your liver. You'll be asked to hold your breath while the biopsy needle is inserted through a small incision in the skin and thrust rapidly into and out of the liver to remove a sample of tissue for lab analysis. You have to hold your breath because the liver must not be moving when the needle goes in, or it could be lacerated. Because the liver is located in the upper abdomen, directly underneath the right diaphragm, the biopsy needle actually passes through the chest cavity. But the needle is inserted so quickly into the liver—for just a second—that most people say the pain isn't severe. The exact method of the biopsy may differ slightly depending on the size of the liver and type of needle used.

Afterward, a bandage will be applied to the site and you'll be asked to lie on your right side. Most hospitals perform liver biopsies on an outpatient basis, keeping patients six hours after the procedure. You will be given pain medication if needed after the procedure provided your blood pressure and breathing are normal. An overnight stay may be necessary if your blood pressure changes, you experience bleeding, or you have any other problem.

About half of patients report no discomfort, but the other half complain of varying degrees of pain. One of the most often reported problems is referred pain in the right shoulder. Acute referred pain may require painkillers.

The lab tests conducted on the tissues may reveal the presence (or absence) of cirrhosis or liver cancer. If you already know you have one of these conditions, the biopsy can help evaluate the progress of the disease and treatment.

THE BENEFITS

Biopsies can help:

- *determine the severity of liver disease (inflammation)*
- *determine the amount of scar tissue (cirrhosis)*
- *clarify the diagnosis if results of blood tests or other exams are confusing*
- *decide on whether to prescribe interferon treatment (most patients with cirrhosis don't respond well to interferon, and those with little liver damage don't need the drug)*
- *screen for liver cancer*

THE RISKS

While the biopsy is currently the best way to determine the amount of liver damage, it's not perfect, and not all doctors believe every patient needs to have a biopsy before treatment. Between 5 to 10 percent of the time, the results of the biopsy underestimate the amount of inflammation or scar tissue in the liver; less than 1 percent of the time the results overestimate the amount of liver damage.

For this reason, some doctors recommend that you have another liver biopsy between one and five years after the first to confirm the original biopsy and to document progression (or lack of it) in the course of the disease. The National Institutes of Health agrees that a series of biopsies is the best way to monitor the progression of chronic hepatitis C.

While liver biopsy is quite safe and unlikely to have complications, it does carry some risks, including:

- *pain (1 in 5 patients)*
- *bleeding (1 in every 500 patients)*

- *puncture of gallbladder, lung, kidney, or intestine (1 in 1,000)*
- *bleeding to an extent that may require transfusions or surgery (1 in 1,000)*
- *death (1 in 5,000)*

The primary risk of liver biopsy is bleeding from the site of needle entry into the liver, although this occurs in less than 1 percent of patients. To reduce the risk of bleeding, your doctor will check how well your blood clots before the procedure. If your coagulation time (prothrombin) is too low or your platelet count is too low, a standard biopsy is not recommended. (However, some patients with bleeding disorders such as hemophilia, which can be temporarily corrected with transfused clotting factors, can be biopsied safely.)

Occasionally, there is a risk that you could have a sudden drop in blood pressure after a biopsy caused by the vagal reflex, not by blood loss. This reaction is caused by the sudden irritation of the peritoneal membrane. If this occurs, you will have slow pulse, sweating, and nausea.

There are less common alternatives to a liver biopsy. In a *laparoscopy,* a doctor inserts a foot-long lighted tube into a small, one-half inch incision in or near the navel to observe the abdominal structures directly. First, the doctor inserts a large needle into the incision to introduce gas into the abdomen. The internal organs are moved away from the abdominal wall by this gas. Then the needle is withdrawn and the laparoscope is inserted in its place. It can be redirected to view and operate on the liver. Instruments may be passed through the lighted tube, or through separate puncture sites, to obtain a tissue sample from several different areas of the liver. If you undergo this procedure, you may be discharged several hours afterward. General, spinal, or local anesthesia may be used.

AUTOIMMUNE HEPATITIS TESTS

Nonroutine blood tests are done when autoimmune hepatitis is suspected. (These might include serum IGS, mitochondrial abs, and antinuclear antibody.) You usually need to ask for your doctor to order these extra tests. In the past, experts thought that autoimmune hepatitis existed only when the patient didn't have any viral forms of hepatitis. Today, experts know that this isn't true in cases of hepatitis C.

Immunological Evaluation Tests

antinuclear antibody (ANA) Indicates possible autoimmune hepatitis

mitochondrial abs Positive in primary biliary cirrhosis and autoimmune hepatitis

rheumatoid factor Positive in autoimmune hepatitis

serum IGS Increased levels in chronic active hepatitis (especially autoimmune hepatitis)

CHAPTER 5

TREATMENT

*W*hile nearly four million Americans are infected with the hepatitis C virus, a new survey shows that less than 25 percent of people with the disease are being treated—mostly because there are few distinctive symptoms that can be recognized.

If you've gotten this far, you've already cleared the first hurdle—you know or you suspect you have the infection. Now you need to think about treatment and understand what you're up against. It's important that you comprehend the nature of this disease; the risk of chronic hepatitis, cirrhosis, and liver cancer; and the availability of treatments. It's also important to weigh the risks and benefits of interferon treatment, especially since there is no solid evidence that treatment will necessarily change the eventual course of the disease. What doctors know right now is that the only treatment for hepatitis C does not cure it or even eradicate the virus—it only suppresses the infection.

As you evaluate your options, you'll need to educate yourself and learn to work together with your treatment team, including your primary care physician, gastroenterologist, and possibly a transplant surgeon. Each year, up to 180,000 more people will be facing these issues as they receive a diagnosis of hepatitis C. Until recently, there wasn't much that could be done to treat the disease.

It's important that you understand there is no cure for hepatitis C. In the few years since the virus has been identified, researchers have been trying to find more and better treatments. Today, the only drug treatment for chronic hepatitis C currently approved in this country by the Federal Drug Administration (FDA) is alpha-2a interferon (Roferon-A) and alpha-2b (Intron) and Infergen (interferon alfacon-I), a consensus interferon. While this treatment is fairly effective, there is still no doubt that this therapy regimen is far from optimal. We just don't have that many effective treatments for any type of viral infection. There is still a great deal of work to be done to determine the best ways to use the drug against HCV.

Interferon is a protein that is naturally produced in your body to fight infection; alpha interferon is an artificially produced copy of the natural protein. The drug, which was first approved for use against chronic hepatitis C in February 1991, both interferes with virus reproduction and stimulates the immune system to fight infections. According to researchers who have reviewed hundreds of studies of hepatitis C, no drug that we know of can eradicate the virus, but treatment with certain interferons can suppress virus replication, reducing and delaying liver damage.

The drug is especially useful because patients with chronic hepatitis C infection do not seem to be able to produce normal amounts of natural interferon on their own. While interferon is used to try to stop the hepatitis C virus from damaging any more of your liver, once your liver is already damaged, interferon can't undo that trauma.

So why isn't everyone rushing out to prescribe this medicine? Interferon is an expensive drug with a variety of side effects, and it's effective at suppressing infection in only about a quarter of the people who take the drug for a year. Moreover, almost everyone who responds to interferon treatment will relapse after discontinuing the medicine and have to be re-treated. In those who do relapse and are re-treated, most will again return to normal ALT levels for up to a year, but it's not clear whether repeated six-month courses of treatment, a long-term maintenance program, or some other schedule is the best plan for continued therapy. What is clear to experts is that long-term re-treatment with a fixed dose is not well tolerated and is associated with frequent fluctuating ALT levels.

Although initial reports suggested that as many as half the people who first responded to interferon did not relapse, it's now clear that only 20 to 30 percent will maintain normal ALT levels for six months to a year. In addition, recent data suggest that relapse occurs even more often than had been previously thought, and many people who appear to have responded and maintain normal ALT levels may actually still have active liver disease. Experts now believe that the goal of chronic viral suppression requires prolonged therapy, re-treatment of relapse, and maintenance regimens.

In any case, the best chance you have to respond to interferon, according to experts, is to be diagnosed early and to undergo an aggressive twelve- to eighteen-month course of interferon. It is imperative to start therapy as early as possible since a longer treatment program appears to lead to better results. Indeed, the FDA extended approval in March 1997 for doctors to use one of the hepatitis C drugs (Intron, or alpha-2b interferon) for up to two years per patient. Researchers had found that this drug, used for the longer period of two years, nearly doubled patients' sustained response rate, compared to just six months of treatment.

It also may be a good idea to use interferon on a daily basis when you first begin treatment, since new research suggests that viral resistance during the early phase of treatment is the major cause of treatment failure. Scientists hope that taking interferon on a daily basis when you first begin treatment will help make you better able to fend off this viral resistance. Studies showed that patients who were treated

Schering's Commitment to Care Program

If you have difficulty paying for Interferon, Schering offers a financial assistance program to help. The program is based on a sliding scale, and the interview for eligibility is done over the phone. You will need to have the following information handy:

- tax forms or pay stubs to verify income

- amount of debt (including rent, mortgage, credit cards, loans)

- amount of savings (if any)

- number of people in household

- doctor's name and address

- treatment protocol (dosage, treatment, length of time)

- when you were diagnosed

To reach the program:
In the United States, dial (800) 521-7157, ext. 147. In Canada, dial (800) 363-3422 (enter 1 for English, 2 for French); when asked for the code, punch in 2000 for the financial assistance line and 0 to speak with a nurse.

with this initial higher dose were less likely to develop cirrhosis four years later, compared to patients treated with less aggressive schedules. The benefits of this more aggressive treatment were especially noticeable in patients with more advanced liver disease, or who had the genotype HCV-1.

Besides hepatitis C, alpha interferon is approved to treat AIDS-related Kaposi's sarcoma and genital warts. Schering-Plough Corp. of Kenilworth, New Jersey, makers of Intron-A, offers a special program for people who can't afford the drug (see Schering's Commitment to Care Program), which can cost in the range of $75 per dose.

HOW INTERFERON WORKS

Most effective when given early in the infection, the drug *temporarily* causes a drop in the liver enzyme levels, and reduces or eliminates the damage to liver cells in about half of those who take the drug for six months. However, up to 60 percent of patients who seem to respond at first will then suffer a relapse (that is, their liver enzymes rise again) within several months after the drug is stopped. Most patients who respond at first but then relapse will respond again if additional treatment is given.

Scientists believe that longer treatments will likely result in longer positive responses. In patients who respond and are treated for six to eighteen months, about 35 to 40 percent have continued normal liver enzymes after the end of treatment.

WHO RESPONDS?

The most important factors associated with a favorable response to interferon are:

- *low levels of virus RNA in your blood before treatment*
- *HCV genotype 3*
- *no cirrhosis*

It appears that the type of infection you have—the genotype—may be very important in the kind of results you get with a specific type of treatment. Unfortunately, genotypes vary considerably not just from country to country, but region to region within a country. This is why studies of different treatment methods are hard to compare, since they may have been treating people with different genotypes who respond differently to interferon. Literally dozens of studies of various interferon dose regimens seem to demonstrate superiority of every conceivable variety of dosing. Since genotypes are so geographically diverse and have significant influence on response to interferon, trials conducted on one continent or even in different regions of a country are not comparable. Instead, studies need to be conducted that compare results from people with similar genotypes and amounts of virus in their blood.

How well you respond to interferon once treatment has begun is usually determined by blood tests your doctor will order from time to time during the treatment program. Recent studies have found that people whose blood levels of virus RNA drop quickly during the first few weeks of treatment will likely have better responses. When your liver tests (ALT) return to normal levels and remain there for at least six months after the treatment is stopped, your doctor will consider this to be a complete and sustained response. Unfortunately, this doesn't always mean the virus has been eliminated from your body. Some people who seem to have responded to treatment no longer have liver inflammation, and their ALT levels are normal—but other tests show they continue to have the virus in their blood.

Ultimately, between 10 and 15 percent of patients have a long-lasting, sustained response to interferon treatment as represented by normal liver enzymes; some of these people will appear to be cured, with no detectable trace of the virus left in their blood.

Those who are going to respond to interferon treatment will do so within two months; therefore, if your condition has not improved by the third or fourth month, your infection will not respond to this round of drug treatment and treatment should be stopped.

If you don't respond the first time, you can be treated again. However, doctors aren't sure how long this second round of treatment should last or what size dose is required for long-term remission in this group.

Still, the issue of what role interferon plays in the course of hepatitis C is not fully understood. Scientists hope that normal liver test results and reduced inflammation in the liver will slow or interrupt the development of progressive liver disease. But the true impact of interferon on the long-term course of chronic hepatitis C is not yet known.

BREAKTHROUGHS

Some patients who appear to respond well at first to interferon treatment and whose ALT levels return to normal within the first few weeks suddenly experience what is known as *breakthrough.* In these cases, a person's ALT levels, which had returned to normal, suddenly begin to rise again, causing what is essentially a relapse in the middle of treatment. These episodes are usually associated with a reappearance of hepatitis C RNA in the blood. Scientists believe that what is really happening is that the virus is becoming resistant to the interferon. No one is sure why this happens, but some suspect it may have to do with changes in the virus itself that make it resistant to treatment.

INTERFERON AND ACUTE HEPATITIS C

In the past, interferon was used only to treat people with chronic hepatitis C. However, there is growing consensus among HCV experts that interferon treatment for people with acute hepatitis C reduces the risk that the infection will become chronic.

Four randomized research studies all showed that some subjects with acute infections responded with either lower ALT levels or hepatitis C RNA in their blood after a four- to twelve-week course of interferon. Although most of these people who responded maintained their good response to treatment, some who responded early on later showed evidence of infection.

Unfortunately, it's not easy to identify people with acute hepatitis C infections, and they are only rarely identified. Acute infection often carries no obvious symptoms, and doctors consider it to be impractical to routinely screen the blood of everybody with identifiable risk factors—especially since 40 percent of hepatitis C patients have no known risk factors.

WHAT THE TREATMENT INVOLVES

Standard treatment as of this moment requires that you get injections three times a week for a year. It's not an easy schedule, and it is expensive (between $2,000 and $5,000 for six months of treatment). You will have to give yourself a needle just below the skin with the same type of needle used by diabetics to give themselves insulin. Your doctor will teach you how to give yourself the shots. Your doctor will also know by the eighth week of treatment whether you are responding; if not, the treatment will be stopped.

Deciding whether or not to take the drug is not always easy, partly because of the cost and also because it can cause flu-like side effects that may be severe. Of course, not every patient experiences these side effects.

Because hepatitis C may not cause any symptoms itself until the very late stages, many people complain that the side effects of inter- feron treatment are far worse than the symptoms of the disease itself. If you are a healthy carrier, choosing treatment is certainly not a clear- cut case: A person who has the virus may feel perfectly healthy and have normal liver tests, and your doctor will probably not be able to predict with any degree of accuracy how the disease will affect you. After all, most people die *with* the disease, not *from* the disease.

Should You Take Interferon?

Because interferon is effective in only a small percentage of patients, it is important that only those people most likely to respond to treat- ment be given therapy. As time goes on and scientists understand more about hepatitis C—especially how different genotypes affect treatment outcomes—the better your own doctor will be able to predict how you will respond to treatment and what the course of your disease will be.

At the moment, what researchers do know is that patients under age thirty-five who have not yet developed cirrhosis have the best response to interferon. Your doctor may recommend alpha interferon treatment if you have had hepatitis for more than six months, your liver enzyme levels (ALT and AST) are more than twice normal, and you haven't drunk alcohol more than twice a week for the past six months.

Alpha interferon appears to work best with patients who:

- *don't yet have cirrhosis*
- *have a hepatitis genotype other than 1*
- *have hepatitis RNA blood levels lower than 2 million/ml*

Unfortunately, your doctor won't be able to predict whether or not you will respond to treatment before you start therapy. However, it may be possible to determine that your disease is too mild to warrant interferon therapy, or that you have other problems that would make interferon treatment unwise for you. A liver biopsy is usually done before treatment to determine the severity of your liver damage and to confirm the presence of underlying disease (see Chapter 4).

Once therapy begins, you will know that the treatment is working if your liver enzyme levels begin to decrease. Ideally, your liver enzymes should drop to within normal levels by the eighth week of treatment. A *sustained response* is defined as liver enzymes remaining normal for six months after treatment stops.

YOU SHOULDN'T TAKE INTERFERON IF . . .

Interferon is not recommended for everyone. For example, interferon often fails to work in people who have hepatitis C but who still have normal ALT levels (liver function test).

It's not a good idea for pregnant women to take interferon. At the present time, little is known about the effect that interferon has on the development of fetal cells.

Interferon and HIV Patients

There is no reason why patients with both HIV and HCV infections should not be considered for treatment with interferon before onset of immunodeficiency. Patients with both infections appear to respond no differently to interferon than do patients who are infected only with HCV, although no study has yet compared their HCV-RNA levels.

Patients infected with both HIV and HCV have an increased risk of liver failure from chronic hepatitis C. The level of virus RNA in the blood increases with full-blown AIDS.

Therefore, you should not take alpha interferon if you think you are pregnant or you are planning on becoming pregnant soon. While you are taking interferon, you must use contraception during treatment and for six months afterward. Since little is known about the effect of alpha interferon on sperm, doctors also recommend that men taking interferon should not try to impregnate their partners while undergoing treatment and for six months afterward.

Other people with hepatitis C may benefit from interferon, but because of their particular medical problems, they should be treated *only in a clinical trial.* This includes those with:

- *fluid in the abdomen (ascites)*
- *bleeding from dilated veins in the esophagus (variceal bleeding)*
- *mental confusion (encephalopathy)*

Other people with hepatitis C and certain diseases or complications are not suitable for interferon at all. This includes people over age sixty or who have:

- *heart, lung, or kidney disease*
- *organ transplants and take prednisone, cyclosporine, or FK-506*
- *history of major depression or taking antidepressants*
- *history of suicide*
- *autoimmune disease (such as diabetes or psoriasis)*
- *a severe drop in white blood cells or platelets*

GENOTYPE AND INTERFERON

Your genotype may also affect how well you will respond to interferon treatment and how serious your disease will become. Most experts believe that infection with type 1 leads to the most aggressive disease, responds poorly to interferon, and recurs more quickly after liver transplant. Type 1b is more aggressive than type 1a.

Another factor that may influence whether you respond well to interferon is the presence of hepatitis C quasispecies. These quasispecies are variations of the same genotype within the same patient that originate from the same infecting virus. Quasispecies may become more diverse over time and may contribute to interferon resistance. (For more information on genotype, see Chapter 2.)

But while genotyping may be useful in determining who may respond better to interferon, experts say it should not be used to determine who is suitable for treatment and who is not. Scientists do not completely understand the full meaning of the genotypes and how individual patients will respond. Much more research needs to be done before experts fully understand the impact of different virus species and their responses to treatment.

SIDE EFFECTS

Numerous side effects have been recorded with interferon. The first dose usually causes the strongest side effects. Within six to eight hours after therapy first starts, you may start to notice flu-like symptoms with fever, chills, and muscle aches. These symptoms may last four to eight hours, but they often disappear as your body gets used to the extra interferon. Some patients find that taking acetaminophen (Tylenol) can help ease discomfort.

Almost everyone feels tired while taking interferon, and most patients have one or more side effects. However, experts say that most side effects are mild to moderate and are tolerated reasonably well. All side effects fade away once the treatment is stopped. Fewer than 10 percent of subjects in research studies have stopped taking interferon because of side effects. Doctors have little idea what the long-term risks are.

COMMONLY REPORTED SIDE EFFECTS

- *flu-like symptoms (chills, fever, malaise, muscle aches, headache)*
- *appetite and weight loss*
- *nausea and vomiting*

- *increased need to sleep*
- *psychological symptoms (irritability, anxiety, depression)*
- *hair loss (mild)*

LESS COMMON SIDE EFFECTS

- *diarrhea*
- *heart palpitations or arrhythmia*
- *insomnia*
- *numbness*
- *skin irritation at site of injection*
- *triglyceride increase*
- *vitiligo*

UNUSUAL SIDE EFFECTS

- *seizures*
- *acute psychosis*
- *bacterial infection*
- *autoimmune disease*
- *pneumonitis*
- *hyperthyroidism or hypothyroidism*

RARE SIDE EFFECTS

- *kidney problems or failure*
- *rashes*
- *optic neuritis*

Of all these side effects, you may find that the most trouble-some problems are the so-called neuropsychiatric side effects—fatigue, drowsiness, lack of initiative, irritability, confusion, apathy, behavioral changes, mood changes, and severe depression. Some patients complain that interferon makes them depressed, and severe depression and suicidal thoughts have occurred even among people who weren't depressed to start with. This is why doctors warn that if you are clinically depressed before you even *start* treatment, you should be evaluated and treated by a mental health expert before taking interferon.

Interferon administration at night can help reduce the frequency of these neuropsychiatric problems, which fade away within several weeks after the end of therapy.

Other side effects that concern doctors include the possibility of the development of thyroid problems in up to 20 percent of patients that may not be reversible after stopping treatment, unless therapy is stopped early. Long-term thyroid replacement in these patients may be required. Still, serious problems with hyper- or hypothyroidism are uncommon.

Because the drug can lower the level of white blood cells and platelets, your doctor will want to take frequent blood tests (at least once a month) to monitor your white blood cells, platelets, and liver enzymes.

It's a good idea to continue working while you are treated and to maintain your regular daily habits. If you have trouble coping with the interferon, you should talk to your doctor about your feelings. Support groups and on-line chat rooms and help lines are helpful to many patients who are taking interferon. (See Appendixes A, B, and C.)

CHILDREN AND INTERFERON

Unfortunately, hepatitis C occurs often among children who received multiple blood transfusions before blood screening for hepatitis C was introduced in 1990. In about 5 percent of cases, youngsters were infected by their mothers before or shortly after birth. The rate at which the infection becomes chronic in these children is not known, but the disease in children appears to be mild.

There are few studies that examine interferon use in children with chronic hepatitis C infection, and interferon is not licensed for use in children under age eighteen. Young children treated with interferon suffer from loss of appetite, weight loss, and growth retardation. Because of these side effects, experts recommend that children under ten not be treated except in the setting of controlled trials. In any case, because the disease is usually mild in children and long-lasting, there is no urgency to treat children since newer treatments may well be developed in years to come.

However, children need to understand that they carry the infection in their blood and that anyone coming in contact with their blood needs to take precautions. Infected teenagers need to understand the risks of drinking alcohol, the possibility of transmitting the infection to others during sex, and the risks of injected drug abuse.

COMBINATION TREATMENTS

The brightest hope for boosting the effectiveness of interferon may lie in combinations with *ribavirin*, according to Douglas Dieterich, M.D., clinical associate professor of medicine at New York University School of Medicine. While other drugs are being tested in combination with interferon, the most promising combination seems to be interferon and ribavirin, which interrupts the ability of the virus to copy itself.

Ribavirin was one of the first antiviral drugs ever discovered. It is approved in the United States in an aerosol form for the treatment of a severe lung infection in infants. Used alone, ribavirin is not very effective against hepatitis C; liver enzymes fall quickly after solo treatment begins, but they often bounce right back within weeks. There is often little change in the amount of virus actually circulating in the blood.

Ribavirin appears to disrupt the process of viral replication by providing a substance that resembles the virus's own enzyme, which is then assimilated by the virus. Scientists hope that by fooling the virus this way, it can't assemble the proper set of genetic material and can no longer replicate.

Ribavirin appears to enhance the effectiveness of interferon when the two are taken together. Initial studies have found that the two drugs in combination may be up to three times more effective than interferon alone. At the moment, Schering-Plough Corp. is studying the effectiveness of a combination of its version of interferon with ribavirin (Rebetol). While the combination of these two drugs has shown promise, according to a panel sponsored by the National Institutes of Health, experts believe the toxicity of mixing interferon and ribavirin needs further study.

It seems that the combination helps to convert some partial responders to complete responders. But it is not clear whether poor responders to interferon alone (people who have high levels of virus RNA in their blood and hepatitis C genotype 1b) will respond any better to this combination.

The main reported side effects of ribavirin include a metallic taste, dry mouth, flatulence, nausea, headache, irritability, fatigue, insomnia, rashes, and myalgia. A mild, reversible anemia is also common when ribavirin is given in doses of 1,200 to 1,600 mg per day. The anemia ends quickly if you take a lower dose or stop taking the drug. At 800 mg per day, ribavirin does not seem to cause anemia.

Despite its complexity, ribavirin is not an expensive drug. A variety of generic imported versions is also available.

Other combination treatments include interferon and a new drug called *Zadazin* (a drug originally isolated from the thymus gland). Zadazin appears to promote maturation of T cells, thereby enhancing the immune system. Tests with this drug showed promise in an Italian study when given together with interferon, but it is still years away from approval in the United States. The long-term benefits of these strategies is at present not known. Interferon combined with *thymosin*

(thymosin alpha 1), a substance associated with the thymus gland and an important part of your immune system, has been yielding promising results. Studies have used synthetic thymosin alpha 1 intravenously against hepatitis C.

Still other combination treatment pairs interferon with *iron reduction therapy* for an effective cure rate of about 75 to 80 percent, according to recent research. This theory is based on the fact that since viruses need iron to replicate, reducing the available iron in the liver should interfere with that reproduction. Adding *cytokines* and other antivirals (such as ribavirin) to the iron reduction method boosts the rate even higher, according to reports published in the *American Journal of Gastroenterology*. While encouraging, this treatment has not yet been approved by the FDA and is still in the early clinical trial stages.

There are also a few trials of *interleukin* (a form of cytokine) used alone. It has been used to treat HIV patients, and a few studies are looking at interleukin as a possible treatment for hepatitis C. Side effects are much the same as for interferon.

Other combination treatments include pairing interferon with *ofloxacin* (OFLX). This antibacterial drug is currently being studied together with interferon after initial studies suggested that ofloxacin might have some antiviral effects. Initial results from Japan suggest that the level of HCV-RNA in the blood decreased after the beginning of combination therapy. In one of every eight patients, the virus RNA completely disappeared. Scientists believe therefore that the combination therapy may be a possible strategy for the treatment of this infection.

The use of the antioxidant *N-acetyl cysteine*, a glutathione source, together with interferon treatment induced a response to interferon in people who had previously failed to respond, according to one pilot study. However, most patients with hepatitis C are not deficient in glutathione, and the therapy is expensive and unpleasant.

Japanese doctors are studying the combination of interferon with *colchicine*, an extract from the bulb of the meadow saffron. Researchers at University of Pisa, Italy, believe that this combination can help people who respond partially to interferon alone become sustained responders the second time around.

While the combination of *pentoxifylline* and alpha-2b interferon reduced ALT levels at first, no long-term benefit has been found. The drug enhances natural interferon production and did reduce levels of tumor necrosis factor, a substance that is associated with liver cell damage.

Combining interferon with bile acid (*ursodeoxycholic acid*) also reduces ALT levels, but it does not seem to eliminate the virus. Likewise, steroids have not been found to be useful against the hepatitis C virus.

Nonsteroidal anti-inflammatory drugs (NSAIDs), when used in combination with interferon, may boost the antiviral effects of interferon through their ability to block prostaglandin synthesis, among other things, but so far this has not been proven.

Other interferons are also being studied, including *consensus interferon* (Welferon) and *beta interferon*.

Other new antiviral medications are currently showing promise, such as *amantadine (Symmetrel)*, used to treat Parkinson's disease and influenza A. The drug, which is much less expensive than interferon, works by interfering with viral replication. Preliminary results showed that 70 percent of the participants achieved at least a partial improvement in their liver function tests. Unlike interferon, amantadine can be taken by mouth.

Other new research targets a form of bursal disease virus (MTH-68/B) that in preliminary trials has a higher response rate and fewer side effects than interferon.

Some scientists in Japan have found that *hemodialysis* appears to reduce the circulating virus in the blood.

ON THE HORIZON

People who don't respond well to these more typical treatments will need newer, different antivirals, several of which are now being developed.

The focus of these new drug investigations centers on enzymes that the virus makes. Some drugs interfere with an enzyme that the hepatitis C virus needs to replicate (*serine protease, helicase* or *polymerase inhibitors*), while others inhibit hepatitis C virus translation.

In recently discovering the enzyme that HCV uses to replicate (called HCV helicase), Schering-Plough researchers used recent technology that allowed AIDS researchers to develop drugs against that disease. Enzymes are catalysts for biochemical reactions in cells. HCV helicase helps hepatitis C make proteins needed to function and uncoils the virus's RNA so it can copy itself to reproduce. At least five companies are working on inhibitors for the enzyme adjacent to helicase.

Scientists are also targeting two other enzymes crucial for protein manufacture; looking at different enzymes in this way could result in many different drugs from which doctors could choose or use in combination against the virus. These drugs are still years away from approval, however. In the meantime, doctors will be relying on alpha interferon to successfully treat some portion of infected patients.

There is a real need for effective antiviral treatments to complement future vaccination programs when these become available. But the lack of any animal model besides the chimp has made developing antiviral compounds difficult.

UNANSWERED QUESTIONS

The long-term outlook for chronic hepatitis C is still not well understood. Scientists do know that it is a slowly progressive disease, with possible transition to cirrhosis in 20 to 50 percent of people; 20 to 30 percent of those will go on to develop liver cancer. There is no proof that treatment with interferon changes these statistics. Experts still can't predict who will develop complications of chronic liver disease and liver failure.

There are still many questions about this treatment. In some studies, women responded better to interferon; obese patients responded less well.

Scientists aren't sure if this is connected to the size of the dose, which is not varied with body weight. Is the gender difference related to iron levels or immune system differences? Or is there really a gender difference at all?

Doctors also aren't sure why patients infected with a single major viral species seem to do better than those with many different quasi-species. Scientists are also baffled by the fact that Egypt has the highest rate of infection of all, where 20 percent of its young and healthy military recruits have HCV. Other tests suggest that infection is more common among heterosexuals than homosexuals.

In the future, doctors hope to have better ways to tell how well patients are responding to treatment so they can fine-tune dose and treatment duration. Researchers hope that ongoing studies will identify these "markers" of response so they can figure out the best way to treat the infection over the long term. It is likely that in the future, doctors will be able to modify treatment according to patient characteristics, such as body size, and the type of infection, such as the specific genotype and how much virus is circulating in the patient's blood. Experts hope that ongoing studies will help determine the best way to manage these infections over the long term.

These new strategies are critical because at present the long-term effects of hepatitis C are troubling. Follow-up of patients who appeared to respond to treatment within ten years showed that many people maintained their response. However, after ten years, there were more reports of late-onset cirrhosis and liver failure. Because the virus may persist indefinitely, some experts believe even patients with no symptoms should be followed on a long-term basis.

ALTERNATIVE TREATMENTS

In addition to more mainstream treatments, there is a variety of alternative treatments for hepatitis C in particular and liver problems in general. If you do choose to explore alternative treatments, it is critical that you do so only with the approval of your doctor. While alternative treatments may seem harmless, it may not be obvious that some herbal medicines and vitamins have unique actions on the liver or on any of the medications you are taking.

If you are participating in a clinical trial, it is imperative that you do not use any type of alternative treatment without first discussing it with your doctor. Such "natural" remedies could influence the results of the study.

MILK THISTLE

One of the most well known "liver detox herbs" is the common plant known as milk thistle (silymarin), which has been used for more than 2,000 years to treat liver diseases. More than 200 studies of the herb in Europe (primarily Germany), South America, and Japan have shown that milk thistle has therapeutic effects in treating chronic hepatitis, among other liver problems.

Native to the Kashmir region of India and Pakistan, the herb has stems and leaves that produce a milky white juice when broken or crushed. Milk thistle, used in traditional medicine since the first century, was enthusiastically endorsed by Roman naturalist Pliny the Elder (A.D. 23–79), who wrote that the plant's juice was good for "carrying off bile." (At that time, "bile" referred to any internal fluid.) By the sixteenth century, British herbalist John Gerard was recommending it for liver problems and fifty years later so did renowned herbalist Nicholas Culpeper. In the nineteenth century, German physicians used a tincture prepared from the milk thistle seeds to treat jaundice and other liver problems.

In 1968 scientists isolated three specific molecules in the milk thistle that were believed to underlie its liver-protective qualities: silibinin, silidianin, and silicristin, now collectively known as silymarin. Because silymarin is not very soluble in water and is poorly absorbed from the digestive tract, researchers produce a medicinal variety processed into tablets or capsules. Most silymarin tablets marketed in the United States come from German sources and contain 70 or 80 percent silymarin.

According to German researchers, silymarin works by strengthening and stabilizing the outer membranes of liver cells, preventing penetration by liver-damaging substances. It also protects liver cells because of its powerful antioxidant action. Antioxidants neutralize cell damage caused by chemically unstable oxygen molecules known as *free radicals*. It also inhibits the action of the enzyme largely responsible for the inflammation of hepatitis and stimulates the production of new liver cells to replace damaged ones. Finally, it seems to be able to boost the liver's ability to filter toxins from the blood.

Taking milk thistle doesn't seem to cause any adverse effects either right away or over the long term. In fact, the plant's young, smooth leaves and stems were once eaten as food in Europe.

While milk thistle extracts are not toxic even when taken for a long time, minor side effects may occur (headache, irritability, and minor stomach upset). It may have a transient laxative effect in some people. Herbalists note it may be used by pregnant and breastfeeding women. To minimize the side effects, herbalists recommend starting with a low dose and increasing it slowly. It typically takes about a month of daily silymarin use to see improvement in hepatitis. Clinicians who prescribe the herb usually recommend that it be taken for one to three months.

Silymarin can be found in herb shops and natural food stores in capsules, liquids, and teas; since silymarin doesn't dissolve well in water, the teas are very weak. The most popular products are standardized extracts of silymarin. Silymarin is safe and nontoxic in doses of 200 to 400 mg; an average dose of milk thistle extract based on the 70 to 80 percent silymarin content is 200 mg. Some herbalists recommend that for the treatment of hepatitis, patients should take 420 mg in three divided doses (140 mg three times a day) for up to nine months, or until improvement is noted. Those who have liver problems and wish to use milk thistle should be monitored by a health care professional.

REISHI MUSHROOMS

The Reishi mushroom is prized by Asian herbalists for its ability to regenerate the liver; it is also believed to modulate the immune system, regulate blood pressure, cleanse the blood, and help the body adapt to the effects of stress.

While that's a tall order for any plant or vegetable, toxicity studies of much higher-than-usual doses (as high as 10 grams per day) have found the mushroom is not toxic to humans and causes no ill effects.

The potency of the Reishi mushroom is usually based on the level of triterpenoids; the more bitter the mushroom, the higher the level of potent substance. Because it is hard and woody, the Reishi mushroom is not eaten but is cut into pieces and brewed as a tea.

Most Chinese herbalists recommend 3 to 5 grams per day brewed as a tea. It is also possible to buy this mushroom as a water and alcohol extract or as a powder.

LICORICE ROOT

True licorice—not the candy, but the root of the plant—contains an active ingredient called glycyrrhizin that is a popular antiviral and is believed by herbalists to be effective in treating viral hepatitis, particularly chronic active hepatitis.

Indeed, an intravenous product containing glycyrrhizin is widely prescribed in Japan to treat hepatitis. Known as Stronger Neo-Minophagen C (SNMC), it was found to be effective in preventing liver cancer in patients with chronic hepatitis C, according to a study published in the April 15, 1997, issue of the journal *Cancer*. The compound, which is comprised of 0.2 percent glycyrrhizin, 0.1 percent cysteine, and 2.0 percent glycine, is an extract of licorice root. Experts suspect that it may protect the liver's cellular membrane, which may explain its ability to lower the blood transamine levels in patients with chronic hepatitis, according to the study by author Dr. Yasuji Arase and colleagues. In his study, Dr. Arase found that after ten years, 7 percent of the group who had been treated with the licorice extract compound developed liver cancer compared with 12 percent of those who had not received SNMC or interferon. The fifteen-year rates were 12 percent for the SNMC group and 25 percent for the others. The authors conclude that long-term administration of the licorice extract can normalize ALT levels and help in protecting against liver cancer.

Available in health food stores as a powder or candy, these products are prepared from the roots and rhizome of European licorice (*Glycyrrhiza glabra*) or other related members of the licorice species— all members of the pea family. The root owes its sweetness and healing power to glycyrrhetinic acid, a compound fifty times sweeter than sugar. It is used widely in Europe in sore-throat formulas, but because of its overpowering sweetness, true licorice is not often used in commercial American candies.

You can find licorice in natural food stores in capsules, lozenges, powders, concentrated drops, tinctures, and extracts. To use, sprinkle a pinch of the powdered herb into hot water or tea. Use for about a week.

Warning: Don't use more than a half ounce (about 3 tsp.) of licorice powder daily over several weeks. Larger or repeated doses of licorice extracts containing glycyrrhizin may cause headaches, lethargy, water retention, high blood pressure, and excess excretion of potassium. Because of these side effects, you should avoid using licorice if you are pregnant or have diabetes, glaucoma, high blood pressure, heart disease, or stroke.

GARLIC

Herbalists believe this natural antiviral can protect the body from infection, detoxify your system, and strengthen blood vessels. Garlic is available in stores as the whole clove, but it is often more easily taken as pills because they don't cause an odor on breath or skin. Garlic is completely nontoxic.

SAINT JOHN'S WORT

This recently popular alternative to antidepressant drugs may also prove helpful in treating hepatitis C, according to some reports. Also known as hypericum, this wild plant has been used for more than 2,000 years to cure a wide variety of diseases. It is believed to have anti-inflammatory, antiviral, and antibacterial properties, and has shown encouraging promise in treating hepatitis C. Exactly how the plant—and its active compound, hypericin—fights viruses isn't understood; it may work by inactivating the virus particles, or by hardening the outer surface of the virus so that it can't infect other cells. It may inhibit the reproduction of viruses, especially if administered in the early stages of disease. Indeed, the herb appears to be a "broad spectrum viricidal agent," according to Daniel Meruelo, Ph.D., professor of pathology at NYU. Researchers from NYU and the Weizmann Institute of Science reported in the *Journal Proceedings of the National Academy of Sciences* that they discovered two substances in Saint John's wort (hypericin and pseudohypericin) that displayed antiviral activity against some retroviruses. While its antiviral activities aren't understood, the chemical structure suggests that the compound may interact with the virus membranes and eventually inactivate the virus. There have been some reports that liver function tests have improved after patients with hepatitis C took Saint John's wort.

THYMIC EXTRACT

This type of alternative treatment, popular in Germany, involves injecting live cells from certain parts of other animals (cattle thymus and shark cartilage are typical) into your blood. While the general idea is an attempt at invigorating the immune system, there are no studies that report on its efficacy in treating hepatitis C.

VITAMINS

Most people have heard that Nobel Prize winner Linus Pauling promoted the use of vitamin C to prevent and treat colds. You may not have known that he also believed the vitamin was an antiviral that could be beneficial in treating hepatitis patients and recommended a minimum of 10,000 mg (or 10 grams a day) up to between 20,000 and 50,000 mg daily (20 to 50 grams). Pure vitamin C pills should be taken three to four times a day; diarrhea can be a problem at higher doses. Other vitamins may also make you feel better, including vitamin B12 and vitamin E, which may help the liver detoxify the blood.

CHAPTER 6

CIRRHOSIS AND HEPATITIS C

*C*irrhosis is a disease of the liver characterized by destruction of liver cells and a permanent breakdown in liver function as a result of infection, poisoning, or alcoholism. About one in five HCV-infected patients will develop cirrhosis of the liver within twenty years, but it's almost impossible to tell beforehand who will be so affected. Cirrhosis is a serious disease because the liver damage is irreversible and there is no cure.

The hepatitis C virus attacks the liver through its cells. As the liver cells die and the thick scar tissue replaces them, more and more of the complicated functions of the liver must be handled by fewer cells. At first, the liver may get bigger in an attempt to compensate for its dying cells, but eventually—as the scarring continues—the liver shrinks. As this happens, it gets harder and harder for the blood to flow to the liver, which slows the liver's processing of nutrients, hormones, drugs, and toxins. Shrinkage also interferes with the liver's production of proteins and other substances.

SYMPTOMS

People with cirrhosis don't usually have many symptoms at first. Early in the course of the cirrhosis, the liver tends to be large, with its cells loaded with fat. The liver feels firm and has a sharp edge that can be felt by a doctor. There may be abdominal pain due to recent, rapid enlargement of the liver. Other early symptoms may include fatigue, weakness, and exhaustion, with a loss of appetite, nausea, and weight loss.

As cirrhosis worsens, the liver becomes harder and smaller as it begins to scar. This change in the liver's structure may lead to permanent impairment of liver function. Fluid builds up in the abdomen and legs. Bleeding is common, and mental processes may slow down.

As liver function declines, the organ produces less protein. As the protein albumin levels drop, water builds up, causing swelling. A decrease in proteins needed to clot blood means patients may bleed or bruise more easily. There is gradual weight loss. Spidery-looking veins resembling bluish-red spiders often appear on the face and trunk.

JAUNDICE

Later stages of cirrhosis also lead to yellowing of the whites of the eyes or skin (known as jaundice) because of the buildup of bile pigments known as bilirubin in the blood. (See Chapter 4.) If the bilirubin is excreted in the urine, your urine will be dark. Some people with cirrhosis experience intense itching due to bile products deposited in the skin. Gallstones often form in those with cirrhosis because not enough bile reaches the gallbladder.

In the late stages of cirrhosis, chronic liver function failure leads to swelling and vitamin K deficiency. Chronic gastritis and gastrointestinal problems can lead to anemia. This anemia, the usual poor appetite and diet by this time, and the poor state of health cause severe fatigue.

Portal Hypertension

Eventually, the liver can become so scarred that blood can't get through the liver at its normal pace because of the scarred obstruction, creating a higher-than-normal blood pressure in the portal vein (the main vein feeding the liver). This pressure causes a condition known as *portal hypertension*. In healthy people, almost all the blood from digestive organs is carried to the liver through the portal vein. If you have cirrhosis, the normal flow of blood is slowed, building pressure to the portal vein into the liver.

As the blood is blocked in the liver, it is forced to back up into the spleen and the gastrointestinal tract. As a result, these organs become chronically congested as well, stagnant with blood that interferes with proper function. This congestion can cause chronic indigestion, constipation, or diarrhea.

Ascites

The problems associated with cirrhosis are not limited to the liver alone. As the liver scars and the blood begins to back up under higher-than-normal tension, this portal hypertension can cause *ascites*, a yellow fluid that accumulates in the abdominal cavity.

The volume of abdominal ascites may reach levels of 10 to 12 liters. This fluid also may build up in the scrotum and the chest cavity, where its presence (combined with the upward pressure of the diaphragm from the abdominal fluid) can affect your breathing. You may lose your appetite because of the stomach distention. If the ascites swell enough and become tense, they eventually can cause a protruding belly button (*umbilical hernia*).

Your doctor can treat ascites and ease your discomfort and breathing by removing the fluid directly from your abdomen with a needle puncture. You'll be placed on a low-salt diet and given diuretics to increase the output of water from your kidneys. If this doesn't control the problem, ascites can be drained internally into the general blood system by running a plastic tube from the abdominal cavity under the skin of the chest into the right internal jugular vein of the neck (called a peritoneovenous shunt of LeVeen).

VARICES

Portal hypertension also may lead to the formation of varices. As the blood into the liver becomes slowed and then blocked, the blood backs up until it bypasses the liver, depleting it of important nutrients. As blood from the intestine tries to find a way around the malfunctioning liver, the liver tries to shunt blood into smaller blood vessels, forcing them to expand. Some of these newly enlarged vessels, called *varices*, may form in the stomach and esophagus and become quite large. Because these vessels were never intended to carry such high pressures and high blood volume, they can rupture and bleed, causing a potentially fatal hemorrhage in the stomach and esophagus.

Esophageal varices are likely to bleed most heavily and lead to the onset of hepatic encephalopathy (see next section) or coma. Because of their location at the end of the esophagus and/or the upper portion of the stomach, bleeding here can be hard to control.

If they are discovered before they burst, varices can be treated on a long-term basis with beta blockers, which lower the blood pressure in the portal vein. Nonsurgical treatment is preferred because of the high death rate surrounding emergency surgery for control of this type of bleeding, and because by this time the patient usually is in poor physical condition due to severe liver dysfunction.

If they do burst, varices can be treated with an endoscope, by placing rubber bands around the varices to tie off the blood. If the bleeding is heavy, a rubber balloon may be inflated at the lower end of the esophagus or upper end of the stomach. These balloons can stop the bleeding by direct pressure. If all else fails, a shunt can be created by inserting a short metal mesh tube through a neck vein into the liver, redirecting part of the blood from the portal vein to another vein in the liver. Another possibility would be to surgically direct some of the blood flow from the portal vein around the liver.

Some doctors believe that bleeding from esophageal varices is a more serious condition than a heart attack. It is certainly a medical emergency; a patient in this condition must be taken to a hospital immediately at the first sign of bleeding—vomiting up blood and/or passing dark stools. Factors that can contribute to this bleeding include lifting heavy objects, coughing or vomiting, straining while having a bowel movement, or sneezing.

HEPATIC ENCEPHALOPATHY

If your scarred and cirrhotic liver has trouble removing toxins from the blood, the toxins may build up in the blood and be carried into the brain. When this happens, your brain becomes poisoned by the toxic elements that are no longer being properly filtered from the blood by the liver. Often, these toxins contain excessive amounts of protein that usually would have been broken down and removed by the liver. As blood levels of these substances increase, they may cause hand tremors and dulled mental function, which could lead to personality changes and even coma (*hepatic encephalopathy*).

If you are in the early stage of toxin buildup in the brain, you may neglect your appearance, feel drowsy and forgetful, have trouble concentrating, or notice a change in your sleeping habits. Your doctor can perform blood tests to determine the ammonia levels—an index of the degree of toxic accumulation.

To treat this problem, your doctor will first stop all drugs that require detoxification in the liver, and then reduce your intake of protein. Restricting the amount of protein in your diet will generally lower the levels of amino acids and ammonia in the bloodstream and brain. Most doctors advise their patients to eat only about forty grams of protein a day (preferably nonmeat protein, such as that in vegetables and milk). Your doctor will probably also prescribe lactulose or neomycin to lower the amino acid production. A dietary supplement rich in certain amino acids (less likely to cause mental impairment) is used at many liver treatment centers.

Diagnosis

Liver function is very complex, so there are many diagnostic tests that can identify cirrhosis. Because you are a hepatitis C patient, your doctor will always be aware of the possibility of the development of cirrhosis, especially if he or she notices visible signs of cirrhosis during a physical exam, such as jaundice, water retention, and spidery blood vessels on your skin (spider nevi). There may be a change in how your liver feels on exam or how large it is.

Based on these findings, your doctor will probably recommend blood tests to find out if liver disease is present. Your doctor may want to take pictures of your liver (computerized axial tomography scan, ultrasound, or radioisotope liver/spleen scan) and order a liver biopsy.

Liver Biopsy

For a definitive diagnosis, your doctor may suggest that a liver biopsy is needed, in which a needle is inserted into the liver to take a sample of tissue. The liver may also be inspected through a laparoscope, a viewing device inserted through a tiny incision in the abdomen. This can reveal the extent and nature of the liver damage.

A liver biopsy can help establish a diagnosis in four out of five cases (for full discussion of the procedure, see Chapter 4). Other than major abdominal surgery under a general anesthetic, your doctor can obtain a liver specimen in one of two ways: a needle biopsy through the skin or a directed biopsy using laparoscopy. Liver needle biopsies are not recommended for anyone with a bleeding disorder, an infection in the right lower lung or in the abdomen near the liver (the needle could carry the bacteria into the liver), abdominal fluid collections, and certain types of jaundice as well as anyone who is uncooperative. Since the patient needs to be observed, needle biopsies are done in the hospital.

A liver biopsy provides the definitive diagnosis, but x-ray and physical exams and several blood tests of liver function are usually performed to monitor the course of the disease. Anyone with cirrhosis is also at risk for hepatic encephalopathy, a group of neuropsychiatric symptoms caused by toxins in the brain that have not been neutralized as they usually are by a healthy liver.

LIVER FAILURE AND LIVER CANCER

Finally, a small percentage of hepatitis C patients with cirrhosis will go on to develop liver cancer, or hepatocellular carcinoma (see Chapter 7). Scientists estimate that about 5 percent of HCV patients with cirrhosis will develop liver cancer over a ten-year period. Some experts believe that some strains of the hepatitis C virus are more virulent than others (particularly type 1b) and more rapidly lead to cancer. Others argue that type 1b might cause more cases of liver cancer because it could be an older virus and is therefore more likely to have progressed in those patients to malignancy.

In any case, liver experts don't yet understand how the hepatitis C virus causes cancer, but it is the leading cause of liver cancer in Japan.

TREATMENT

Unfortunately, there is no specific treatment for cirrhosis, and once the cirrhosis occurs, it cannot be reversed even if the underlying inflammation is stopped. Research suggests that interferon does not have much effect on cirrhosis caused by hepatitis C, but those few patients who do respond tend to go into remission. Other studies suggest that the diminished response to interferon in patients with cirrhosis may be partly overcome by combining interferon with ribavirin.

Otherwise, your doctor will try to treat and prevent symptoms and complications. A no-salt diet and water restrictions can help deter fluid retention. This diet needs to be followed carefully, since even small boosts of salt in the diet may produce considerable swelling. Your doctor also may prescribe diuretics to help remove fluid from your system. If you have any signs of confusion or encephalopathy, your doctor may also advise a low-protein diet, together with vitamins K, A, and D.

For itching complaints, doctors may prescribe the drug cholestyramine. Because this drug can interfere with the absorption of other drugs, it should be taken separately. You should not drink any alcohol or take any other drug that is broken down and eliminated by the liver. If you absolutely must use one of these medications, your doctor may be able to adjust the dosage to ease trauma to your already ailing liver. If your cirrhosis is severe enough, your doctor may consider a liver transplant (see Chapter 9).

CHAPTER 7

LIVER CANCER

If you have hepatitis C infection, odds are that you won't develop either cirrhosis or liver cancer. However, a small percentage of people will go on to experience more serious liver disease, and doctors have no way of predicting who will be so affected.

What scientists do know is that hepatitis C infection is a major risk factor for the development of liver cancer (hepatocellular carcinoma) around the world. In the United States, about 5 percent of hepatitis C patients with cirrhosis will develop liver cancer and about 1 percent of all hepatitis C patients will probably one day be diagnosed with this condition. The problem is even more widespread in southern Europe and Japan.

Other studies have found that it is possible for some hepatitis C patients—especially those who have the virus genotype 1b—to have liver cancer without first developing cirrhosis. In the United States, liver cancer usually takes many years to develop, although in a few patients it has appeared in as little as five years from the onset of HCV infection.

The precise way that hepatitis C causes liver cancer is not known. Unlike the hepatitis B virus, hepatitis C does not become a part of the genome of liver cells. It is more likely, scientists say, that liver cancer occurs together with, or as a result of, inflammation and regeneration associated with liver injury due to chronic hepatitis. Most cases of HCV-related liver cancer occur in combination with cirrhosis; this suggests that cirrhosis is really the risk factor for liver cancer, not the HCV infection itself.

Many scientists suspect that some cirrhotic nodules that grow larger than others (called *adenomatous hyperplasia*) are the precursor to liver cancer. On the other hand, other doctors believe that altered liver cells may appear in between these nodules and these could grow to become the adenomatous hyperplasia—and eventually, liver cancer.

RISK FACTORS

Obviously, not all people with hepatitis C infection—and not all people with both HCV infection and cirrhosis—will go on to develop liver cancer. You are considered to be at higher risk for developing liver malignancy if you are older, male, and have more severe underlying liver disease. Other risk factors include drinking too much alcohol and having both hepatitis B and C infections at the same time. Your viral genotype may be important in the development of liver cancer as well, although early suggestions that infection with genotype 1b carries a greater risk of liver cancer haven't been confirmed in larger studies.

Viral load—the level of actual virus in your blood—is associated with the severity of liver disease, but no clear link has been established between blood levels of the virus and liver cancer.

You can see by all this information that your liver cancer risk can't really be accurately determined. What experts do know is that about 20 percent of patients with HCV infection will develop cirrhosis over a ten-year period. Among those with established cirrhosis in screening programs, between 3 and 4 percent per year develop liver cancer (at least for the first four or five years of screening). What this means is that twenty years after infection, scientists can predict that a small percentage of patients with chronic hepatitis C can be expected to develop liver cancer.

TREATMENT

At present, partial removal of the liver or a total liver transplant offers the best hope for prolonged survival. Unfortunately, partial removal for liver cancer is associated with a high recurrence rate (about 25 percent per year). While the intent is to cure the disease, in fact patients with cirrhosis who undergo this procedure usually have only a 33 percent survival rate after five years. On the other hand, liver transplant for patients with small, inoperable tumors have a five-year survival rate of between 60 and 80 percent (for more information on transplants, see Chapter 9).

Scientists are studying other treatments currently available, including ethanol injection, interferon therapy, and lipiodolization.

ETHANOL INJECTION (PEI)

PEI involves an injection of *pure* ethanol into the tumor under radiologic guidance to kill the tumor. This procedure appears to be effective, is inexpensive, and is widely available. It is believed to be equally as effective as tumor removal for local tumor control. This type of under-the-skin injection is usually recommended for patients with tumors that could be removed, but who don't want to undergo the surgery or who are poor surgical risks (often because these patients have advanced liver disease). This type of treatment is not appropriate if you have liver ascites, or lesions on the surface of the liver.

Interferon Therapy

Some researchers suggest that progression to liver cancer can be halted or at least slowed down by treating the underlying hepatitis C infection. For example, recent Japanese studies have suggested that patients with cirrhosis caused by chronic HCV have a significantly lower risk of liver cancer if they are treated with alpha interferon. This improvement in risk occurs both in those patients whose hepatitis C infection responded to interferon therapy and those who did not. (For more information, see Chapter 5.)

Lipiodolization (Targeted Chemotherapy)

Scientists are presently studying the effectiveness of *lipiodolization*, the use of lipiodol together with a chemotherapeutic agent concentrated within the tumor. This type of targeted chemotherapy provides a better response than regular systemic chemotherapy. However, there are frequent side effects including fever, nausea, abdominal discomfort, and rarely, hair loss.

Prognosis

Typically, once a patient develops liver cancer, the prognosis is poor. Patients usually die within six months after diagnosis, but if it is detected early enough it may respond better to treatment and cure. Small tumors have the potential for cure, but large tumors are associated with a poor prognosis; most of these patients die within the first year.

CHAPTER 8

OTHER COMPLICATIONS OF HEPATITIS C

*T*he most serious problems you'll
have to worry about with hepatitis
C are cirrhosis and liver cancer. There is
one particular liver problem that doesn't
happen often, but which can be very
serious when it does occur.

In a few rare cases, the symptoms of hepatitis C develop quickly
and become very severe. This condition is known as *fulminant
hepatitis*, or fast-progressing hepatitis, and it is fatal up to 80 percent
of the time. Fulminant hepatitis can cause the kidneys to fail, the
liver to shrink as cells die, and within a short time, a fatal coma.
The development of this condition requires immediate medical
attention.

In addition, the hepatitis C virus can attack cells in the rest of
your body. Most often, the virus affects the skin, joints, kidneys, blood
vessels, and thyroid gland, causing a variety of autoimmune diseases,
skin symptoms, and other problems.

AUTOIMMUNE DISEASES

Hepatitis C chronic infection is associated with a wide range of autoimmune diseases (conditions where the body develops antibodies that attack the person's own tissues). This condition can cause treatment-related problems, since immune supplements such as interferon may cause additional problems in patients with autoimmune symptoms.

About one out of ten people with chronic hepatitis C have antibodies to their own thyroid gland, which can lead to a sluggish thyroid (hypothyroidism). A host of other autoimmune diseases are also linked to hepatitis C, including cryoglobulinemia, autoimmune hepatitis, and symptoms of rheumatoid arthritis.

Between a third and a half of patients with chronic hepatitis C also suffer with *cryoglobulinemia*, a disorder in which abnormal proteins in the blood damage the skin, nervous system, and kidneys. Only about 20 percent of people with hepatitis C and cryoglobulinemia develop symptoms, which include mild fatigue, joint pains, or itching. Once in a while, someone with the disorder will develop Raynaud's disease, an inflammation of the blood vessels that can cause numbness of hands and feet, purple skin lesions, or redness from intermittent constriction and dilation of the blood vessels.

Hepatitis C-related cryoglobulinemia is not a condition that occurs soon after a person becomes infected with the virus; it usually appears in patients who have developed cirrhosis or who have had hepatitis C for many years. However, those people with higher amounts of virus in the blood don't seem to have any higher risk of developing cryoglobulinemia. Fortunately, cryoglobulinemia does not affect how a patient will respond to interferon, and some patients who have inflammation notice an improvement as their liver tests improve while taking interferon.

Hepatitis C virus is one of the major causes of *autoimmune hepatitis*, a very serious condition that leads to cirrhosis within only three years in more than 80 percent of patients. In this condition, some patients have been successfully treated with interferon despite the fact that interferon is not generally recommended in patients with autoimmune symptoms.

Finally, the debilitating autoimmune condition known as *rheumatoid arthritis* may also be associated with hepatitis C.

SKIN LESIONS

Hepatitis C is associated with a variety of skin disorders. It may lead to *lichen planus*, a group of small, itchy, irregular, flat-topped red bumps on the skin, covered with a network of fine gray lines. The bumps appear most often on the wrists, shins, lower back, and genitals. In the mouth, lichen planus looks like a white, net-like plaque; it may also appear as mouth ulcers. It can be treated with a steroid mouth rinse or antifungal medication.

Hepatitis C may be associated with the development of *spider nevi*, small capillaries that you can see on the surface of your skin. Less than ten is considered normal; more than ten spider nevi is an indication of chronic liver disease. Spider nevi are typically found only above the waist, especially on the face, neck, upper back, chest, upper arms, and shoulders.

Hepatitis C is a major cause of *porphyria* throughout the world and is the most common trigger of porphyria in people who are predisposed to that condition. Porphyrins are a group of compounds primarily produced in bone marrow that play an important role in many chemical reactions in the body; they are later converted to bile pigments, primarily in the liver. It is believed that *porphyrinuria* (increase of porphyrins in the urine) may be caused by chronic liver disease. *Porphyria cutanea tarda*, a rare deficiency of a liver enzyme essential for cellular metabolism, may lead to blisters and ulcers on sun-exposed skin that can then turn dark or bruised. Hair may grow on the forehead, cheeks, or forearms, and the urine may turn pink or brown. Topical sunscreens won't prevent the skin lesions, but avoiding alcohol and giving blood to lower excess iron levels may help. Alternatively, chelation therapy (taking medication that binds to iron) may help. Chloroquine (an anti-malarial drug) removes a toxin by-product of the enzyme deficiency and may help.

LYMPHATIC DISEASE

While researchers understand that HCV often infects the lymphatic system, it is not believed to cause lymphatic disease very often. However, occasionally this infiltration may lead to a type of cancer known as B cell non-Hodgkin's lymphoma. Scientists in Italy have reported that 34 percent of patients with this type of cancer also have hepatitis C.

COMPLICATIONS OF CIRRHOSIS

Some complications of hepatitis C are associated with the development of cirrhosis (scarring) of the liver (more fully discussed in Chapter 6). These cirrhotic complications include hepatic encephalopathy (changes in the brain as a result of advanced liver disease) with loss of memory, disorientation, untidiness, and muscular tremors.

CHAPTER 9

LIVER TRANSPLANTS

*L*iver transplants are the final, last-ditch effort to save seriously damaged livers ravaged by hepatitis C and cancer. It's the most common reason for all liver transplants in the United States today. It's important to understand that while a transplant may take care of cancer, it won't cure hepatitis. Because the hepatitis C virus can live in cells outside the liver, the virus simply moves into the newly transplanted organ in a matter of weeks or months.

The good news is that the second time around, the virus's attack on the liver is often much less severe. Despite the fact that viral infection persists in more than 95 percent of hepatitis C patients who have had liver transplants, the reported five-year survival rate is 60 to 80 percent. However, the fact that hepatitis C is a chronic infection suggests that as years go on, these patients may experience more problems than patients without hepatitis C infection.

When the virus does mount another attack on the liver, most of the time it does not seriously damage the new organ. While it is occasionally possible for the infection to return to such a ferocious degree that the transplanted liver fails, this is uncommon. Only about 20 percent of patients face this problem.

It's fortunate that few livers fail within three years of transplantation (only about 5 percent) because retransplantation is not nearly as successful; more than 50 percent of retransplants fail.

The first liver transplant was performed in 1963, but in those early days of transplant medicine, few of the patients with transplanted livers lived more than a few months. However, since 1981 the outcome for liver transplant patients has been steadily improving; today more than three-quarters of these patients are alive a year after surgery, due in part to improved surgical techniques, better methods of preserving donated organs, and better postoperative care. An important development has been the use of the immunosuppressive drug cyclosporine.

When should you consider a liver transplant? It's not an easy answer, but in the early stages of hepatitis C infection it is not usually necessary. When drug treatment can't halt the progression of the virus and the liver has become irretrievably damaged, either through cancer or cirrhosis, your only option may be a liver transplant.

The survival rate for transplantation in patients with small but inoperable liver tumors is between 60 and 80 percent after five years— better than any other mode of therapy. However, the decision to do a transplant is not a simple one. You and your doctor will want to consider how fast your disease is progressing, whether you have developed complications of liver failure, and the results of some lab tests. At some transplant centers, it is possible to have a liver transplant even if you are infected with both hepatitis B and C.

Consider the pros and cons of a liver transplant.

PROS

- *removes both detectable and undetectable cancer*
- *cures the underlying cirrhosis*
- *offers best chance for long-term survival*

CONS

- *expense*
- *liver shortage*
- *danger of HCV reinfection of organ*
- *immunosuppressive drugs may speed up the growth of tumors*

Transplants for end-stage liver cancer (stages III and IV) are more controversial and are not currently recommended by the National Institutes of Health. In one study, 54 percent of patients with end-stage liver cancer lived for three years after receiving chemotherapy; however, this treatment remains experimental.

No one knows whether a transplanted liver will last a lifetime or not. The longest reported survivor has been twenty-five years after transplant; ten years is common. Since doctors have been able to diagnose hepatitis C only since 1990, there are not many long-term studies of survivors after liver transplants to consider.

WHO IS ELIGIBLE?

The operation may be offered to anyone with potentially fatal liver disease. Most likely candidates are people with HCV who are under age sixty. People with alcohol problems, however, are considered to be poor risks for transplantation, since the recurrence rate and potential damage are so high. Previous surgery in and above the upper abdomen may make liver transplantation difficult or risky.

THE TECHNIQUE ITSELF

Liver transplants are the most expensive and probably the most difficult single-organ transplants possible. On a national average, they cost about $250,000 per patient. Because liver transplantation is not an easy surgical technique, requiring between eight and ten hours of surgery, it's available at only a few large medical centers. One of the most successful programs is located at Stanford University Medical Center, where more than 87 percent of patients survive more than one year and more than 83 percent live at least three years after they receive new livers—the highest patient survival rates for liver transplants in the nation. Because of the team's extensive experience and meticulous surgical techniques, nearly a third of its patients don't require any transfusion of blood or blood products. (In general, liver transplant patients need twelve to twenty units of blood during the operation.)

After the surgery, you'll spend several days in intensive care, and then between two and four weeks in a regular hospital room before release. The first six weeks after your surgery, you'll have frequent tests to monitor your liver function and whether your new organ is being rejected. Once the liver is transplanted, remember that it can be ambushed fairly quickly—within weeks—by the HCV virus. The drugs you take to suppress rejection of the new organ seem to make your new liver vulnerable to the infection.

Your routine follow-up will include monthly blood tests and blood pressure checks. Keep in mind that the drugs you take to head off rejection will increase your susceptibility to infection. If you're taking cortisone-like drugs, they will cause some fluid retention and a puffy face, and can worsen diabetes and osteoporosis. Cyclosporine and tacrolimus can cause high blood pressure and possible kidney damage—but the risks can be lowered by monitoring your drug levels.

What your doctor is concerned about at this point is failure or rejection. Keep in mind that there can be degrees of liver failure, and it's possible that your liver may not be functioning perfectly even if you feel fine. If rejection does begin, it can be treated with drugs to reverse the problem.

The risk of rejection is most severe within the first few weeks after surgery. For this reason, the dosage of your anti-rejection drugs will be higher at first and then gradually decrease. By six months post-surgery, you will need only relatively low doses of these drugs as a maintenance program for the rest of your life.

You should begin to feel healthier right away if your new liver is functioning well, and you'll be back doing regular exercise within six to twelve months. The rest of your life should return to normal. In fact, several women who have had liver transplants went on to have successful pregnancies and deliveries.

TAINTED LIVERS

Because donated organs are in short supply, sometimes a patient who desperately needs a new liver can accept one from a donor who was HCV positive, but whose liver had not yet been damaged. Doctors in this case would biopsy the liver and if it was found to be fairly healthy, it could be transplanted into a patient who also has HCV. What doctors hope in this case is that the liver might have been from someone who was recovering from HCV and who had only lingering antibodies to HCV—or who perhaps had false-positive tests for HCV. But even if the donor had active HCV, an unharmed liver from that donor could still extend your life considerably. Keep in mind that many people with HCV live long, healthy lives without ever developing cirrhosis or liver cancer, and the donated liver could well have come from someone in that situation.

AFTERCARE

After the transplant, you will need numerous liver biopsies in the early weeks to months following surgery to accurately diagnose whether the new liver is being rejected or whether other problems have developed.

Of course, it's wise to try to keep this liver as healthy as possible. Avoid alcohol, liver-toxic drugs, pollution, pesticides, caffeine, nicotine and cigarette smoke, illegal drugs, and any other substance that is hard on your liver.

You will need lifelong therapy with immunosuppressive drugs to prevent rejection of the new organ, but at low maintenance levels.

CHAPTER 10

WHAT TO DO IF YOU HAVE HEPATITIS C

It's important to realize that chronic viral hepatitis only rarely interferes with lifestyle or employment. Although you may feel tired, especially if you are taking interferon treatments, many patients find this fatigue comes and goes. Neither prolonged bed rest nor strenuous exercise affects the disease, so you should maintain your normal level of activity.

FINDING A DOCTOR

It's important to find a specialist who has experience in treating hepatitis C. The symptoms of hepatitis can be mimicked by a host of other illnesses, including chronic fatigue syndrome, autoimmune illnesses, cancer, and so on. A hepatologist specializes in diseases of the liver and might be the best choice, followed by a gastroenterologist (specialist in digestive diseases) or an infectious disease specialist.

It's also a good idea to consider joining a hepatitis support group near your home; these groups can offer names of helpful specialists. Alternatively, you can contact the American Liver Foundation (ALF) for a list of doctors near you. If you need more information about hepatitis, ask your doctor, nurse, or pharmacist. You can also contact the ALF at (800) 223-0179. The ALF is the only national voluntary, nonprofit health organization dedicated to treating, curing, and preventing hepatitis and other liver and gallbladder diseases through research and education. See Appendix A for information about organizations that deal with liver issues; see Appendix B for a listing of Internet sites about hepatitis C.

MAINTAINING YOUR HEALTH

Doctors offer a number of suggestions to maintain your health:

1. EAT A HEALTHY DIET.

While there isn't any magic food that will cure hepatitis, it is true that nutrition and liver function are intricately related—and some processes are better understood than others. Since everything you eat, breathe, and absorb must eventually be either refined or detoxified by your liver, it makes sense to pay special attention to your diet—especially if you have hepatitis. Doctors recommend regular, well-balanced meals and avoiding excessive weight gain.

If you have cirrhosis as well as hepatitis C, getting the right amount of protein can be tricky. People with cirrhosis need a balanced diet rich in protein, between 2,000 and 3,000 calories a day to allow liver cells to regenerate; too little protein can interfere with healing. But excessive protein will raise the level of ammonia in the blood too much. For this reason, check with your doctor for guidance on the correct amount of protein if you have cirrhosis. Doctors can also prescribe two drugs (lactulose and neomycin) to control blood ammonia levels. You will want to avoid uncooked shellfish, which can be very dangerous for hepatitis C patients with cirrhosis.

If you have cirrhosis and an uncomfortable buildup of fluid in your abdomen (ascites) or swelling in various parts of your body, you may get relief by eating less salt and avoiding most high-sodium prepared foods, such as canned soups and vegetables, cold cuts, dairy products, mayonnaise, and tomato products.

A Diet to Keep Your Liver Healthy

For a healthy liver, try to eat these foods:

- fresh fruits and vegetables

- whole grains

- fish

- legumes

- organic chicken

It's best to avoid these foods:

- fried foods

- spicy foods

- foods high in refined sugar or alcohol

- stimulants (coffee and cola drinks)

- alcohol

2. DON'T DRINK TOO MUCH ALCOHOL.

It's a good idea to stop drinking alcohol if you have hepatitis C because scientists think alcohol boosts the activity of the hepatitis C virus and increases liver damage. No one knows if there is a safe amount of alcohol that hepatitis C patients can drink; if you really want to drink, most doctors recommend you limit alcohol to no more than one drink per day. Alcohol should be completely avoided by alcoholics and anyone with cirrhosis. While an occasional alcoholic beverage may be safe for some people with hepatitis C, abstinence is still recommended by most experts during treatment, since any amount of alcohol use on a daily basis is potentially harmful.

Japanese studies have found that drinking lots of alcohol (more than three drinks per day) interferes with the effectiveness of interferon therapy in habitual drinkers with chronic hepatitis C; this effect can be reversed once the person stops drinking. Studies also suggest that drinking alcohol may be related to the development of hepatitis C infection itself, and it may be partly responsible as well for the development of both cirrhosis and liver cancer among heavy-drinking hepatitis C patients.

3. STOP SMOKING.

If you have hepatitis C and you smoke cigarettes, studies show that you are at higher risk for developing liver cancer than if you didn't smoke. Since your liver must detoxify the poisonous components of the smoke, you'll do yourself a favor if you can cut down or eliminate smoking completely.

4. AVOID STREET DRUGS.

If you're struggling with hepatitis C, it's a good idea not to stress your liver any more than it already is. For this reason, it's important not to use any street drugs during the acute phase of hepatitis C infection, so your liver has a chance to repair itself. If you can't stop using drugs, remember that purer forms of drugs are better—so methadone would be better than street heroin, for example. Because your affected liver has more problems in detoxifying your body during hepatitis C, you will also run a greater risk of overdosing (especially on alcohol and benzodiazepine tranquilizers).

5. TRY TO MAINTAIN A POSITIVE, HOPEFUL ATTITUDE.

You shouldn't underestimate the impact of stress on your immune system. Recent research at Hershey Medical Center shows that stress may influence how sick you can get from a viral illness and how long it will take to recover. Consider a variety of stress-busters:

- Relax. *A good way to avoid stress is to learn how to relax. Your pulse and breathing will slow, blood pressure fall, and muscles relax. You can try books, relaxation tapes, or a meditation course. As little as twenty minutes a day can bring significant relief.*
- Reframe! *This technique is a way to change the way you look at things in order to feel better. There are many ways to interpret the same situation.*
- Cut down on caffeine. *You will feel more relaxed if you substitute decaf or caffeine-free beverages. You'll feel less jittery, more relaxed, and less nervous. You'll have less heartburn, and you'll sleep better.*
- Don't forget to sleep. *It may seem obvious, but sleep is an important way to reduce stress. If you're tired, you can't cope very well with stressful situations.*
- Pace yourself. *Monitor your stress level; if you start to feel as if you're going to blow your top, take a deep breathe and step back. Give yourself permission to make the time to enjoy your life.*
- Build a support system. *Remember that a problem shared is a problem halved. It's not easy to handle a chronic disease. Try to create a solid support structure of family and friends with whom you can discuss your fears and concerns. Check out some hepatitis C support groups, Internet chat rooms, newsletters, and so on. If at any time you find yourself without a support system, consider seeking out a counselor so that you have someone with whom to share your emotions.*

Are You Depressed?

Depression has been associated with hepatitis C. Surely it's not easy living with this little-understood chronic disease with its uncertain etiology, unclear diagnosis, and ill-defined prognosis. Treatment with interferon as well may make some people more depressed than usual. It's critically important that you seek help if you do start feeling down. How do you tell the difference between the blues and a full-blown clinical depression? Take this test to find out if you're depressed:

- Are you often sad or anxious?

- Do you often feel empty inside?

- Do you feel helpless, guilty, or worthless?

- Do you think there's little hope for a cure for hepatitis C?

- Have you given up?

- Have you lost pleasure in participating in activities you used to enjoy?

- Do you have less energy?

- Is your memory not as sharp as it used to be?

6. BE PREPARED FOR A LACK OF UNDERSTANDING.

You may be shocked to find people treating you differently after your diagnosis. Some may think of hepatitis as a "junkie's disease"; others may be afraid of somehow catching your infection. If your condition begins to interfere with your life, people may not be so ready to offer you support.

7. DRINK PLENTY OF WATER.

If you're taking interferon, it's important to drink as much plain water (not tea, coffee, or soda) as you can tolerate in order to ease the severity of side effects and to head off possible kidney infections caused by not getting enough water.

8. GET VACCINATED.

If you have hepatitis C, you should be vaccinated against both hepatitis A and B as well. Having one infection will not protect you from getting a second, and there is evidence that having more than one infection can worsen the condition of your liver.

9. BEWARE OF TOXINS.

If your liver is already under attack, you'll want to avoid other substances that are harmful to this organ. Avoid paint fumes, nicotine, chemical preservatives, harsh cleaners, and air pollution.

10. MAINTAIN YOUR LEVEL OF ACTIVITY.

Since neither bed rest nor strenuous activity affects the outcome of hepatitis C, you should maintain your normal level of activity.

- Do you have trouble concentrating?

- Are you restless and irritable?

- Do you have sleeping problems?

- Has there been a change in your interest in sex?

- Do you eat more or less than you used to?

- Do you often find yourself thinking about death?

If you answered "yes" to more than five questions, especially if these feelings lasted more than two weeks or are interfering with your normal life, you should seek professional help.

CHAPTER 11

PREVENTION

*While there is as yet no vaccine
that can prevent the spread
of hepatitis C, screening of the nation's
blood supply has decreased the risk
of disease from blood transfusions from
10 percent in the 1970s to less than
1 percent today.*

Since little can be done in the way of treating hepatitis for most people, the goal is really to prevent any other individuals from transmitting the infection. Moreover, becoming infected with one type of hepatitis will not protect you from getting another kind. There is also evidence that becoming infected with both hepatitis B and C is linked to developing a much more severe, dangerous case of hepatitis.

Moreover, it is unclear whether the presence of HCV antibodies will protect you from being reinfected with HCV. In other words, if you appear to have recovered from an HCV infection, doctors are not positive that you can't get it again, based on inconclusive studies with chimps. This uncertainty could be due to the constantly mutating state of the HCV virus and the large variety of genotypes and subspecies.

Still, as in other blood-borne diseases, you may be able to avoid transmitting hepatitis C by taking proper precautions. Take these precautions if you have hepatitis C:

DISPOSE OF BLOOD-SOAKED ITEMS CAREFULLY

You should dispose of any blood-soaked items yourself. For example, if you cut yourself while shaving, or if you have a nosebleed, you should be the one to discard the tissues. Open wounds should be covered, and instruments that may be contaminated by blood—razors or toothbrushes, for example—should not be shared.

DON'T SHARE NEEDLES OR ANY OTHER DRUG-RELATED EQUIPMENT

If you have hepatitis C, it is important to notify anyone who has shared intravenous drug equipment with you and to urge them to seek medical care.

DON'T DONATE BLOOD OR PLASMA, SPERM, TISSUES, OR ORGANS

The hepatitis C virus can be easily transmitted to any organ transplant recipient who obtains a contaminated organ. All potential organ donors are tested for hepatitis C before their organs are used in transplant operations.

If you found out about your infection in some way other than by giving blood, and you've given blood in the past, you should notify your local blood donor clinic, and tell them when and where you last gave blood. You should not donate blood, plasma, semen, or organs. You should also inform your dental and medical health providers so they can take proper precautions when treating you.

Don't Share Personal Care Items

Don't share razors or toothbrushes with anyone. As a courtesy, you should let any health care professional (doctor, nurse, dentist, podiatrist, etc.) who cares for you know that you have hepatitis C.

However, you don't need to use separate bathroom facilities or eating utensils, such as cups, bowls, silverware, and so on.

Practice "Safer" Sex

The rate of transmission by sexual contact is considered to be low enough that doctors don't believe condoms are necessary within monogamous relationships, but some experts still recommend that all patients with HCV infection use barrier contraception. Recommendations in this area are controversial.

Recent estimates suggest that the average couple having an average frequency of sexual activity would have to live together for more than 600 years before the susceptible partner would acquire HCV infection. However, it is not a

To Help Prevent Liver Disease

It's not likely that a healthy liver will prevent infection with hepatitis C, but certainly a healthy immune system can help fight off any infection and minimize the seriousness of infections that do occur. To keep your liver healthy and your immune system strong:

- Don't consume more than two alcoholic drinks a day.
- Be careful when mixing several drugs (especially alcohol with certain medicines).
- Avoid taking medicines you don't need.
- Avoid exposure to industrial chemicals whenever possible.
- Maintain a healthy, balanced diet.
- Consult your doctor if you notice any symptoms of liver disease.
- Avoid too much junk food fats (french fries, fried chicken, doughnuts, etc.).
- Don't drink too much coffee (carcinogenic hydrocarbons are produced during roasting, and dark roasts are the worst).

- Don't smoke. Tobacco and marijuana smoke contain toxic benzoapyrene, polycyclic aromatic hydrocarbons, cyanide, acetaldehyde, tars, acrolein, and so on that the liver must detoxify. Virtually all components of smoke are known to be at least mildly liver toxic.

- Avoid exhaust and air pollution.

- Think twice about birth control pills (in some cases, just two or three weeks of use have ruined the ability of the liver to detoxify naturally produced estrogen).

- Avoid pesticides—certain pesticides such as DDT, aldrin, chlordane, lindane, and so on can cause chronic liver damage, even at body levels measured in parts per billion, and tend to accumulate in body fat over time.

- Avoid certain drugs—Dilantin, phenobarbitol, Nizoral are a few potentially liver-toxic drugs.

- Avoid chronic steroid abuse, which is linked to serious liver damage.

- Avoid long-term contact with gas, diesel fuel, motor oil, and degreasing agents, all of which are liver toxic and may be absorbed through the skin or inhaled.

good idea to have sex during menstruation or to have anal sex in order to minimize the possibility of infection.

Although sexual transmission is extremely rare, you should advise any potential partner of your infection. If you have sex with more than one partner, you should practice safe sex (use a latex condom).

Of course, it is not necessary to limit expressions of affection; hug your family often. They won't catch the infection from you.

COVER OPEN SORES

Since the virus is in your blood, you need to be careful not to allow anyone else to come in contact with your blood. Cover all open sores or other breaks in your skin.

VACCINES

At the present time, there are no vaccines available to prevent hepatitis C infection, and scientists don't see much chance of one in the near future because the HCV mutates at a very fast rate. Scientists thus have problems establishing stable cultures of the virus in which to develop the vaccine. Shots of gamma globulin after a person has been stuck with a contaminated needle do not seem to work.

It appears that people can't develop an immunity to HCV as they can to other viruses. Researchers believe this is because the virus constantly changes to new forms of the original virus that had caused the body to produce antibodies.

Making the development of a vaccine even more difficult is the fact that more than six strains of HCV exist, depending on the geographic region in which you live.

ORGANIZATIONS

American Liver Foundation
1425 Pompton Ave.
Cedar Grove, NJ 07009
(888) 4-HEPUSA or (973) 256-2550
The only national, nonprofit health agency dedicated to preventing, treating, and curing hepatitis through research, education, and support groups.

CDC Hepatitis Hotline
(404) 332-4555
Voice mail allows you to request faxed information.

Global Hepatitis Support Network
511 Ave. of the Americas
Ste. 148
New York, NY 10011
      or
130 Prim Rd.
Ste. 511
Colchester, VT 05446
(802) 655-2579
A nonprofit organization providing support to hepatitis C patients.

Hepatitis C Foundation, The
A grassroots organization founded and run by volunteers who offer information, personal support, and referrals, together with a twenty-four-hour 800-number help line. The foundation provides emotional and psychological support, information, and referral sources. It is launching an extensive campaign to promote awareness of hepatitis C and to support research and development to create additional treatments in the hope of finding a cure.

Hepatitis C Foundation (political action/education committee activist group)
The arm of the Hepatitis C Foundation and an organizing venue for HCV-related activism. People can join as members of the HCF-PAEC activist group and participate in any campaigns and projects. The goal is to work toward better research funding; patient support and public, patient, and physician education programs; improved treatments; and a cure for hepatitis C. The group is organized and run by volunteers who have hepatitis C.

Hepatitis Foundation International
30 Sunrise Terrace
Cedar Grove, NJ 07009
(800) 891-0707 or (201) 239-1035
Provides updated information on new diagnostic measures and treatments, referral to physicians, and access to a telecommunications network of patients with similar ailments.

National Digestive Diseases Information Clearinghouse
(301) 654-3810
An informational group that provides facts on hepatitis C.

Well Spouse Foundation, The
P.O. Box 28876
San Diego, CA 92198
(619) 673-9043 or (914) 357-8513
Support group that provides emotional support to spouses of the chronically ill, advocates insurance changes for respite and long-term care, and produces bimonthly newsletter.

APPENDIX B

ON-LINE INTERNET SITES

American Association for the Study of Liver Diseases
A page of interest to liver disease specialists with information on association membership, meetings, publications, and courses.
http://hepar-sfgh.ucsf.edu/

American Liver Foundation
Frequently asked questions (FAQs) are cross-referenced for in-depth help; patients can obtain updates on treatment and research.
http://liverfoundation.org

American Share Foundation
The web's largest transplant-related site, with links to other helpful information.
http://www.asf.org/

Ask Emaliss (Hep C Info and Support)
A free monthly on-line magazine that provides a place for submitting personal questions and receiving answers. Some of the Q&As are published in the "shared voices" section. Also included: editorials, tests and treatment information and experiences, letters to the editor, activist information and news, and more.
http://soli.inav.net/~webbsite

BACafe
Provides support and information about hepatitis C, with websites, FAQs, information for the newly diagnosed, and HCV kids page.
http://www.flash.net/~twb/BACafe/

Canadian Liver Foundation, The
Home page for the foundation with lots of helpful information.
http://www.liver.ca

CDC Emerging Diseases Page
Information about emerging diseases (including hepatitis C).
http://www.cdc.gov/ncidod/EID/eid.htm

CenterWatch Clinical Trials Listing Service
Site that allows you to sign up for E-mail notification of every new clinical trial investigating hepatitis C.
http://www.centerwatch.com

CenterWatch Patient Notification Service
Site that notifies patients seeking information about clinical trials and new drugs approved by the FDA for hepatitis C.
http://www.centerwatch.com/PATEMAIL.htm

Chronic Hepatitis Answering Page
Send in your HCV questions for Dr. Brillanti to answer.
http://llovrworld.compuserve.com/homepages/SBrillanti_2/

Columbia University Diseases of the Liver
Site with lots of information about liver diseases.
http://cpmcnet.columbia.edu/dept/gi/references.html

Current Papers on Liver Disease
Site with information on liver disease.
http://cpmcnet.columbia.edu/dept/gi/references.html

Elaine's Hepatitis C Resource Page
Resources for information about hepatitis C, including all the latest medical research as well as a personal touch.
http://www.geocities.com/HotSprings/2630/index.html

Focus On: Hepatitis C International
Helpful site with lots of good information.
http://pages.prodigy.com/hepc/

HCV Support and Info
Several pages of web links, chat rooms and schedules, personal stories, and local support groups.
http://members.aol.com/hcv3020458/Index.html

Hepatitis and Liver Disease Referral Network
Listing of prominent hepatologists.
http://www.arens.com/hepnet/

Hepatitis A, B, and C: Questions and Answers
A brief page describing the differences between various types of hepatitis, with information on prevention and treatment.
gopher://gopher.uiuc.edu/oo/UI/CSF/health/heainfo/diseases/contag/hepa

Hepatitis C Foundation
Information, personal support, and referrals.
http://www.hepcfoundation.org
E-mail: hepatitis_c_foundation@msn.com

Hepatitis Foundation International
Resources, information update, support, and links to books and other products.
http://cpmcnet.columbia.edu/dept/gi/hcpint.html

Hepatitis C Information and Support
Lots of information on recent research, including discussions about interferon, liver biopsies, and milk thistle therapy.
http://planetmaggie.pcchcs.saic.com/hepc.html

Hepatitis C Society
Home page for the Hepatitis C Society in Canada with information about HCV.
http://web.idirect.com/~hepc/

Hepatitis C (Spanish)
Information presented in Spanish about hepatitis C.
http://www.chasque.apc.org/freno/hepcespa.html

Hepatitis C Virus
Professional journal site with detailed information on hepatitis C.
http://www.ccm.Isumc.edu/bugbytes/bb-v1n13.htm

Hepatitis Education Project
Nonprofit corporation providing educational materials and support; also publishes a quarterly newsletter.
http://www.halcyon.com/jevo/HEP/

Hepatitis Haven
Site offering directory, links, transplant information, drug information resources, and singles personal ads for people with HCV.
http://www.tiac.net/users/birdlady/hep.html

Hepatitis Information Network (Hepnet)
Designed for both medical professionals and patients who are looking for current information on viral hepatitis A through G. Also offers quizzes, original papers, daily news, worldwide educational symposiums, and more.
http://www.hepnet.com

Hepatitis Mutual Support
A place to go for support and links to many informational sites on hepatitis, liver diseases, cirrhosis, interferon, and other home pages about hepatitis.
http://members.aol.com/VikkiSM/hepage.html/

Hepatitis WebRing
Home page for the Hepatitis WebRing dedicated to providing a simple yet exciting and efficient means of locating websites with information pertaining to hepatitis.
http://www13.pair.com/jude/hepring

Hep C Connection
Helpful site with lots of information about hepatitis C.
http://www.hepc-connection.org

HEP Education Project
Nonprofit corporation providing education, materials, and information about support groups.
http://www.scn.org/health/hepatitis/

Hep Kids
Interesting place for kids whose loved ones have hepatitis C.
http:home.att.net/nandit/

Hepnet
See Hepatitis Information Network.

Infection Control for Long-Term Care
Links and many infection control topics, including hepatitis and AIDS.
http://web.infoave.net/~dtalbott/

Land of Waz Hepatitis Info

Hepatitis informational site with many places to get help, including a Java enabled health chat box.
http://www.asan.com/users/wazzie/wizpage2.htm

Nashville Hepatitis C Coalition

Home page for a group dedicated to providing information and support to hepatitis C patients, families, and friends.
http://members.aol.com/HEPPER/NashvilleHepC.html

National Institutes of Health

Home page for the NIH with information on hepatitis.
http://www.nih.gov/

National Institute of Allergy and Infectious Diseases

Home page for the NIAID with information about hepatitis.
http://www.niaid.nih.gov/

National Institute of Diabetes and Digestive and Kidney Diseases

Home page for the NIDDKD with information about hepatitis.
http://niddk.nih.gov/NIDDK_HomePage.html

Peppermint Patti's Junk Drawer

Information on hepatitis, with the latest edition of the hepatitis C FAQs. Contains on-the-spot search engines and is frequently updated with new information and sites, including information on fibromyalgia, chronic pain, disability, and coping.
http://www.alaska.net/~clotho/

Ribavirin

Page with information about the drug ribavirin.
http://www.aidsinfonyc.org/pwahg/info/riba.html

Schering-Plough (manufacturers of Intron-a)
Home page for the makers of interferon.
http://www.hep-help.com

UNOS Website (United Network for Organ Sharing Transplants Information)
Offers detailed information on organ transplants.
http://www.ew3.att.net/unos

USER GROUPS/MAILING LISTS

HCV Activist Mailing List

This list is concerned with letter writing, political action, and reform in connection with hepatitis C research and funding. To subscribe, type in the body of the E-mail message—SUBSCRIBE HCV-ACTIVIST—and send the message to:
majordomo@statsrus.com

Hep C Forum Mailing List

A mailing list for patients with hepatitis C. To subscribe, send an E-mail message to majordomo@lists.vossnet.co.uk and type in the body of the message—SUBSCRIBE HEPC. Or visit the forum's website at:
http://village.vosnet.co.uk/c/crina/maillist.htm

Hepatitis Newsgroup

A lively newsgroup for sharing information, research news, and experiences.
USENET sci.med.diseases.hepatitis

HEPV-L

An active mailing list for patients with chronic HCV who share information and stories. A good place to share experiences. To subscribe, type in the body of the E-mail message the words—SUBSCRIBE HEPV-L <YOUR FULL NAME>—and send the message to:
listserv@sjuvm.stjohns.edu

NEWSLETTERS

Focus: On Hepatitis
Quantum Media Group
130 Prim Rd.
Ste. 510
Colchester, VT 05446
(802) 655-2715
National newsletter devoted to hepatitis C.

Hepatitis Weekly
Subscription-based information service that gathers the latest news, research, and journal articles on all varieties of hepatitis, from A to G, together with article abstracts and breaking news.
http://www.holonet.net/homepage/1h.htm

Hep-C ALERT!
A dynamic and quickly growing nonprofit hepatitis activist and advocacy organization, with a "hot topic" page.
http://www.hep-C-alert.org/

Hep C BC
A directory of Internet resources for hepatitis C, with links to hepatitis C support groups and mailing lists, alternative medicine, hepatitis C

Society of Canada and British Columbia chapters, medical journals, medical sites, news, research, clinical trials, transplants, information gathering, and Canadian government sites.
http://www.geocities.com/HotSprings/5670

Hep C Connection
1714 Poplar St.
Denver, CO 80220
(303) 393-9395
$10/year ($1/issue)
Helpful newsletter for HCV patients with the latest research and treatment information, news of conferences, information about support groups, letters, and so on.

Progress
A quarterly consumer newsletter published by the American Liver Foundation.

GLOSSARY

abscess   A localized formation of pus in a cavity caused by the disintegration or displacement of tissues due to bacterial infection.

acute   A term used to describe a condition that occurs abruptly or that runs for only a short time. It is the opposite of chronic.

albumin   A protein found in the blood that can be measured to assess how effectively your liver forms proteins. A problem in synthesizing protein could mean you have liver damage. Normal albumin levels are between 35 to 50 grams/liter.

alkaline phosphatases   A type of blood test used to diagnose liver disease. Levels are increased in various forms of hepatitis, cirrhosis, and liver cancer.

amino acids   A component of protein. The body produces many amino acids; those it needs but can't synthesize are known as essential amino acids, and must be obtained through diet.

anemia   A condition characterized by a reduced number of red blood cells, amount of hemoglobin, or amount of blood.

antibody   A protein of the immune system that counteracts or eliminates foreign substances known as antigens.

antigen   A substance foreign to the body that triggers the formation of antibodies.

arrhythmia   Irregular heartbeat.

ascites   An accumulation of excess fluid within the abdominal cavity often seen in chronic hepatitis C.

autoimmune response   The reaction of your body against its own tissues that are incorrectly perceived as foreign substances. This triggers the body to produce antibodies against its own tissues.

bile   Bitter-tasting fluid produced by the liver and temporarily stored in the gallbladder before being released into the small intestines. In the small bowel, bile facilitates the digestion of fats.

bilirubin   Orange to yellow pigment in bile that is the result of the breakdown of hemoglobin. Too much bilirubin produces jaundice and is a sign of liver damage.

biopsy   Removal of a tissue sample from your body to diagnose disease.

CBC   Abbreviation for complete blood count.

cholesterol   Fatty substance synthesized in the liver and found in the blood, brain, liver, and bile, and as deposits in the walls of blood vessels.

chronic   A term that describes a persistent, lingering, or recurring condition.

chronic fatigue syndrome   A disorder characterized by extreme weakness and exhaustion and persistent apathy and depression. Many hepatitis C patients have been diagnosed with this syndrome.

cirrhosis   A condition where normal tissue is replaced by hardened scar tissue; cirrhosis of the liver is found in severe alcoholics and in chronic hepatitis C patients. It may be caused by toxins such as alcohol, or as a result of infection.

diabetes mellitus   A disorder characterized by high levels of sugar (glucose) in the blood. Diabetes mellitus may be caused by a failure of the pancreas to produce enough insulin, or by the body's resistance to the action of insulin.

dialysis   A technique of removing waste and toxins from the blood, used primarily when the kidneys malfunction or after a drug overdose.

DNA (deoxyribonucleic acid)   A substance found in the nucleus of cells that carries genetic and hereditary information.

esophagus   Tube that connects the throat with the stomach.

fatty liver   The abnormal buildup of triglycerides in the liver that can cause appetite loss and stomach discomfort.

fulminant   Refers to a disease that develops quickly and lasts a short time, usually ending in death.

gallbladder   Sac located under the liver that stores bile secreted from the liver and then released into the small intestine.

gamma globulin   A protein found in the blood that helps fight infections.

gastrointestinal tract   The stomach and intestines.

gene   Structure within a chromosome that is responsible for inheritance of a particular characteristic.

genotype   A virus strain with a distinct genetic makeup.

globulin   A category of simple blood proteins of which antibodies are formed.

glutathione   An amino acid important in keeping cells healthy that is often deficient in hepatitis C patients.

glycogen   Stored form of sugar.

HCV   Abbreviation for hepatitis C virus.

hemoglobin   A red pigmented protein that contains iron and is found in the red blood cells. Hemoglobin carries oxygen to and removes carbon dioxide from body tissues.

hepatic   Pertaining to the liver.

hepatic calculi   Stones in the biliary tract or solely in the liver; also found in liver cysts.

hepatic coma   A syndrome characterized by slow or rapid onset of bizarre behavior, disorientation, lethargy, and coma that seems to be caused by a buildup of toxins in the brain due to liver failure.

hepatic encephalopathy   A serious complication of advanced liver disease caused by toxins in the brain (including ammonia) that results in personality changes and impaired intellectual ability.

hepatic failure, fulminant   A clinical syndrome caused by extensive liver tissue death that may lead to a progressive encephalopathy and death.

hepatologist   Physician who specializes in liver disease.

histamine   The active agent of allergic reactions that occur when excessive amounts of histamine are released to combat an invading foreign substance in the body.

HLA type   Abbreviation that refers to human leucocyte antigen, a genetically determined regulator of the immune response. HLA type is related to the odds of a patient recovering from hepatitis C infection.

hyperglycemia   A condition in which too much sugar is present in the blood.

hypoglycemia   A condition in which blood sugar falls below normal amounts.

immunity   State of being resistant to a disease (especially an infectious one).

immunization   Introduction of antigens into the body in very small amounts in order to stimulate the development of immunity.

immunoglobulin   A protein that can act as an antibody.

infection   A condition in which the body is invaded by a microorganism, such as a virus.

infectious   The ability to transmit a disease.

inflammation   A tissue's reaction to injury from infection or irritation, causing swelling, pain, heat, and redness.

interferon   A type of protein that is released in response to the presence of antigens (invading substances). Interferons inhibit the development of viruses and host cells. Initially developed to treat cancer, they are now produced synthetically and used to treat HCV.

jaundice   Yellowing of the skin and eyes due to higher-than-normal levels of bilirubin in the blood. In hepatitis, excess bilirubin in the blood is the result of the liver's inability to metabolize bilirubin due to damage from infection.

LDH   Abbreviation for lactic dehydrogenase; very high levels of this in the blood indicate cancer.

liver   Largest internal organ in the body, and the site of many metabolic functions. These include producing bile, neutralizing poisons, synthesizing proteins, and storing glycogen and certain minerals and vitamins.

myalgia   Muscle pain.

myalgic encephalomyelitis   See chronic fatigue syndrome.

N-acetyl cysteine   A chemical that may protect the liver and attack viruses. It is currently being studied as a hepatitis C treatment in combination with interferon.

NK   Abbreviation for natural killer cell, a type of immune cell.

nonsteroidal anti-inflammatory drugs (NSAIDs) Medications used to reduce inflammation that aren't cortisone-based.

PCR The abbreviation for polymerase chain reaction, a type of test used to assess HCV infection and identify viruses.

portal hypertension An impairment of flow in the portal vein, which supplies the liver, causing rising pressure within the portal system. This leads to enlargement of the spleen and development of enlarged veins (varices) in the esophagus and stomach. Portal hypertension occurs in more than two-thirds of people with cirrhosis of the liver.

protein One of many complex nitrogen compounds, made up of amino acids. Proteins are essential for the growth and repair of tissue.

prothrombin A chemical substance found in circulating blood that interacts with calcium salts to form thrombin, a step in the process of blood clotting.

prothrombin time The time it takes for prothrombin to form thrombin, a step in the process of blood clotting. A prothrombin time of more than five seconds indicates fulminant liver failure.

relapse Recurrence of disease or symptoms after apparent recovery.

remission Absence of symptoms.

resection Partial surgical removal of an organ or tissue.

spleen The organ located to the left and just in front of the stomach that stores and sometimes manufactures blood cells.

thrombin An enzyme that is part of the process of blood coagulation.

thyroid gland　An endocrine gland that helps control the body's rate of function and contributes to maintaining a balance between calcium in the blood and bones.

varices　Distended blood vessels associated with cirrhosis.

viral load　A measure of the amount of virus present in a patient.

virions　Individual virus elements.

virus　Tiny organism that causes disease.

REFERENCES

Aach, R. D., C. E. Stevens, F. B. Hollinger, J. W. Mosley, D. A. Peterson, P. E. Taylor, R. G. Johnson, L. H. Barbosa, and G. J. Nemo. 1991. Hepatitis C virus infection in post-transfusion hepatitis. An analysis with first- and second-generation assays. *New England Journal of Medicine* (Nov 7) 325(19):1325–9.

Abuaf, N., F. Lunel, P. Giral, E. Borotto, S. Laperche, R. Poupon, P. Opolon, J. M. Huraux, and J. C. Homberg. 1993. Nonorgan specific autoantibodies associated with chronic C virus hepatitis. *Journal of Hepatology* (Jul) 18(3):359–64.

Aiyama, T., K. Yoshioka, M. Takayanagi, K. Iwata, A. Okumura, and S. Kakumu. 1995. Serum HCV-RNA titer at the end of interferon therapy predicts the long-term outcome of treatment. *Journal of Hepatology* (Nov) 23(5):497–502.

A-Kader, H. H., and W. F. Balistreri. 1993. Hepatitis C virus: implications to pediatric practice. *Journal of Pediatric Infectious Disease* (Oct) 12(10):853–66; quiz 867.

Akahane, Y., M. Kojima, Y. Sugai, et al. 1994. Hepatitis C virus infection in spouses of patients with type C chronic liver disease. *Annals of Internal Medicine* 120:748–52.

Alberti, A. 1991. Diagnosis of hepatitis C. Facts and perspectives. *Journal of Hepatology* (May) 12(3):279–82.

———. 1997. Retreatment with interferon. *NIH Consensus Development Conference on Management of Hepatitis C* (Mar).

Alberti, A., L. Chemello, P. Bonetti, et al. 1994. Treatment with interferon(s) of community-acquired chronic hepatitis and cirrhosis type C. *Journal of Hepatology* 17(suppl 3):123–6.

Alberti, A., L. Chemello, D. Cavalletto, A. Tagger, A. Dal Canton, N. Bizzaro, G. Tagariello, and A. Ruol. 1991. Antibody to hepatitis C virus and liver disease in volunteer blood donors. *Annals of Internal Medicine* (Jun 15) 114(12):1010–2.

Alberti, A., G. Morsica, L. Chemello, et al. 1992. Hepatitis C viraemia and liver disease in symptom-free individuals with anti-HCV. *Lancet* 340:697–8.

Alberti, A., P. Pontisso, L. Chemello, G. Fattovich, L. Benvegnu, F. Belussi, and M. S. De Mitri. 1995. The interaction between hepatitis B virus and hepatitis C virus in acute and chronic liver disease. *Journal of Hepatology* 22(1 Suppl):38–41.

Alemy-Carreau, M., J. P. Durbec, J. Giordanella, S. Rousseau, G. Blanc, D. Monges, M. Perreard, J. R. Harle, P. J. Weiller, and A. Gerolami. 1996. Lack of interaction between hepatitis C virus and alcohol in the pathogenesis of cirrhosis. A statistical study. *Journal of Hepatology* (Nov) 25(5):627–32.

Allander, T., A. Gruber, M. Naghavi, A. Beyene, T. Soderstrom, M. Bjorkholm, L. Grillner, and M. A. Persson. 1995. Frequent patient-to-patient transmission of hepatitis C virus in a hematology ward. *Lancet* (Mar 11) 345(8950):603–7.

Allison, M., and P. R. Mills. 1996. Screening asymptomatic people at high risk for hepatitis C. The case against. *British Medical Journal* (May 25) 312(7042):1349–50.

Allison, M., T. Wreghitt, C. R. Palmer, and G. J. Alexander. 1994. Evidence for a link between hepatitis C virus infection and diabetes mellitus in a cirrhotic population. *Journal of Hepatology* (Dec) 21(6):1135–9.

Alter, H. J. 1997. Blood donors with hepatitis C. *NIH Consensus Development Conference on Management of Hepatitis C* (Mar).

———. 1995. To C or not to C: these are the questions. *Blood* (Apr 1) 85(7):1681–95.

Alter, H. J., M. Gallagher, T. T. Morris, et al. 1997. Acute non A-E hepatitis in the U.S. and the role of hepatitis G virus infection. *New England Journal of Medicine* 336:741–746.

Alter, H. J., Y. Nakatsuji, et al. 1997. The incidence of transfusion-associated hepatitis G virus infection and its relation to liver disease. *New England Journal of Medicine* 336:747–754.

Alter, H. J., R. H. Purcell, J. W. Shih, J. C. Melpolder, M. Houghton, Q. L. Choo, and G. Kuo. 1989. Detection of antibody to hepatitis C virus in prospectively followed transfusion recipients with acute and chronic non-A, non-B hepatitis. *New England Journal of Medicine* (Nov 30) 321(22):1494–500.

Alter, H. J., R. Sanchez-Pescador, M. S. Urdea, et al. 1995. Evaluation of branched DNA signal amplification for the detection of hepatitis C virus RNA. *Journal of Viral Hepatitis* 2:121–32.

Alter, M. J. 1997. Epidemiology of hepatitis C. *NIH Consensus Development Conference on Management of Hepatitis C* (Mar).

———. 1991. Hepatitis C: a sleeping giant? *American Journal of Medicine* (Sep 16) 91(3B):112S–115S.

———. 1994. Transmission of hepatitis C virus—route, dose, and titer [editorial]. *New England Journal of Medicine* (Mar 17) 330(11):784–6.

Alter, M. J., P. J. Coleman, W. J. Alexander, et al. 1989. Importance of heterosexual activity in the transmission of hepatitis B and non-A, non-B hepatitis. *Journal of the American Medical Association* 262:1201–5.

Alter, M. J., R. J. Gerety, L. A. Smallwood, R. E. Sampliner, E. Tabor, F. Deinhardt, G. Frosner, and G. M. Matanoski. 1982. Sporadic non-A, non-B hepatitis: frequency and epidemiology in an urban U.S. population. *Journal of Infectious Disease* (Jun) 145(6):886–93.

Alter, M. J., S. C. Hadler, F. N. Judson, et al. 1990. Risk factors for acute non-A, non-B hepatitis in the United States and association with hepatitis C virus infection. *Journal of the American Medical Association* 264:2231–5.

Alter, M. J., H. S. Margolis, K. Krawczynski, F. N. Judson, A. Mares, W. J. Alexander, P. Y. Hu, J. K. Miller, M. A. Gerber, R. E. Sampliner, et al. 1992. The natural history of community-acquired hepatitis C in the United States. *New England Journal of Medicine* (Dec 31) 327(27):1899–905.

American Liver Foundation. 1996. Getting hip to hep: What you should know about hepatitis A, B & C. *American Liver Foundation.*

———. Statement on hepatitis C. 1997. *American Liver Foundation* (March 25).

American Medical News. 1995. Government looks at blood supply safeguards. *American Medical News* (Nov 6).

Ampurdanes, S., E. Olmedo, M. D. Maluenda, X. Forns, F. X. Lopez Labrador, J. Costa, J. M. Sanchez Tapias, M. T. de Anta, and J. Rodes. 1996. Permanent response to alpha-interferon therapy in chronic hepatitis C is preceded by rapid clearance of HCV-RNA from serum. *Journal of Hepatology* (Dec) 25(6):827–32.

Andreone, P., C. Cursaro, A. Gramenzi, A. Buzzi, M. G. Covarelli, L. Di Giammarino, R. Miniero, V. Arienti, M. Bernardi, and G. Gasbarrini. 1996. A double-blind, placebo-controlled, pilot trial of thymosin alpha 1 for the treatment of chronic hepatitis C. *Liver* (Jun) 16(3):207–10.

Angelico, M., C. Gandin, E. Pescarmona, M. Rapicetta, C. Del Vecchio, A. Bini, E. Spada, C. D. Baroni, and L. Capocaccia. 1995. Recombinant interferon-alpha and ursodeoxycholic acid versus interferon-alpha alone in the treatment of chronic hepatitis C: a randomized clinical trial with long-term follow-up. *American Journal of Gastroenterology* (Feb) 90(2):263–9.

Arai, Y., K. Noda, N. Enomoto, K. Arai, Y. Yamada, K. Suzuki, and H. Yoshihara. 1996. A prospective study of hepatitis C virus infection after needlestick accidents. *Liver* (Oct) 16(5):331–4.

Arase, Y., H. Kumada, K. Chayama, A. Tsubota, I. Koida, K. Ikeda, S. Saitoh, T. Matsumoto, and M. Kobayashi. 1994. Interferon retreatment of nonresponders with HCV-RNA-positive chronic hepatitis C. *Journal of Gastroenterology* (Jun) 29(3):299–304.

Ascher, N. L., J. R. Lake, J. Emond, and J. Roberts. 1994. Liver transplantation for hepatitis C virus-related cirrhosis. *Hepatology* (Jul) 20(1 Pt 2):24S–27S.

Atrah, H. I., F. A. Ala, and D. Gough. 1994. Blood exchanged in ritual ceremonies as a possible route for infection with hepatitis C virus. *Journal of Clinical Pathology* (Jan) 47(1):87.

Bach, N., and H. C. Bodenheimer, Jr. 1992. Transmission of hepatitis C: sexual, vertical or exclusively blood-borne? *Hepatology* (Dec) 16(6):1497–9.

Bain, V. 1997. Therapy for hepatocellular carcinoma. *The Hepatitis Information Network HomePage* (Jun 18).

Balart, L. A., R. Perrillo, J. Roddenberry, F. Regenstein, K. S. Shim, Y. S. Shieh, B. Taylor, S. Dash, and M. A. Gerber. 1993. Hepatitis C RNA in liver of chronic hepatitis C patients before and after interferon alfa treatment. *Gastroenterology* (May) 104(5):1472–7.

Ballmer, P. E., J. Reichen, M. A. McNurlan, A. B. Sterchi, S. E. Anderson, and P. J. Garlick. 1996. Albumin but not fibrinogen synthesis correlates with galactose elimination capacity in patients with cirrhosis of the liver. *Hepatology* (Jul) 24(1):53–9.

Bar-Shany, S., M. S. Green, R. Slepon, and E. Shinar. 1995. Ethnic differences in the prevalence of anti-hepatitis C antibodies and hepatitis B surface antigen in Israeli blood donors by age, sex, country of birth, and origin. *Journal of Viral Hepatology* 2(3):139–44.

Barton, A. L., B. F. Banner, E. E. Cable, and H. L. Bonkovsky. 1995. Distribution of iron in the liver predicts the response of chronic hepatitis C infection to interferon therapy. *American Journal of Clinical Pathology* (Apr) 103(4):419–24.

Bayraktar, Y., D. H. Thiel, and A. Gurakar. 1996. Hepatitis C and the controversies it creates relative to liver transplantation and autoimmune hepatitis. *Hepatogastroenterology* (Jul-Aug) 43(10):873–81.

Benvegnu, L., D. Cavalletto, M. G. Ruvoletto, and A. Alberti. 1991. Specificity and patterns of antibodies to hepatitis C virus in hepatocellular carcinoma [letter]. *Hepatology* (Nov) 14(5):959. Comment on: Hepatology 1990 (Sep) 12(3 Pt 1):589–91.

Benvegnu, L., G. Fattovich, F. Noventa, F. Tremolada, L. Chemello, A. Cecchetto, and A. Alberti. 1994. Concurrent hepatitis B and C virus infection and risk of hepatocellular carcinoma in cirrhosis. A prospective study. *Cancer* (Nov 1) 74(9):2442–8.

Benvegnu, L., P. Pontisso, D. Cavalletto, F. Noventa, L. Chemello, and A. Alberti. 1997. Lack of correlation between hepatitis C virus genotypes and clinical course of hepatitis C virus-related cirrhosis. *Hepatology* (Jan) 25(1):211–5.

Bernstein, D., K. R. Reddy, L. Jeffers, and E. Schiff. 1995. Canities and vitiligo complicating interferon therapy for hepatitis C. *American Journal of Gastroenterology* (Jul) 90(7):1176–7.

Bird, G. L., E. Spence, K. J. Hillan, R. N. MacSween, D. Frame, P. Yap, B. Dow, F. McOmish, and P. R. Mills. 1995. Genotypic variation, clinical, and histological characteristics of chronic hepatitis C detected at blood donor screening. *Journal of Viral Hepatology* 2(5):261–5.

Blum, H. E. 1994. Does hepatitis C virus cause hepatocellular carcinoma? *Hepatology* (Jan) 19(1):251–5.

Boker, K. H., G. Dalley, M. J. Bahr, H. Maschek, H. L. Tillmann, C. Trautwein, K. Oldhaver, U. Bode, R. Pichlmayr, and M.P. Manns. 1997. Long-term outcome of hepatitis C virus infection after liver transplantation. *Hepatology* (Jan) 25(1):203–10.

Bonkovsky, H. 1997. Other options for treatment of hepatitis C. *NIH Consensus Development Conference on Management of Hepatitis C* (Mar).

Booth, J. C., G. R. Foster, U. Kumar, R. Galassini, R. D. Goldin, J. L. Brown, and H. C. Thomas. 1995. Chronic hepatitis C virus infections: predictive value of genotype and level of viremia on disease progression and response to interferon alpha. *Gut* (Mar) 36(3):427–32.

Bortolotti, F., A. Tagger, P. Cadrobbi, C. Crivellaro, F. Pregliasco, M. L. Ribero, and A. Alberti. 1991. Antibodies to hepatitis C virus in community-acquired acute non-A, non-B hepatitis. *Journal of Hepatology* (Mar) 12(2):176–80.

Bortolotti, F., R. Giacchino, P. Vajro, C. Barbera, C. Crivellaro, A. Alberti, G. Nebbia, L. Zancan, L. De Moliner, A. Bertolini, et al. 1995. Recombinant interferon-alfa therapy in children with chronic hepatitis C. *Hepatology* (Dec) 22(6):1623–7.

Bresci, G., G. Parisi, S. Banti, and A. Capzia. 1995. Re-treatment of interferon-resistant patients with chronic hepatitis C with interferon-alpha. *Journal of Viral Hepatology* 2(3):155–8.

Bresee, J. S., E. E. Mast, P. J. Coleman, M. J. Baron, L. B. Schonberger, M. J. Alter, M. M. Jonas, M. Y. Yu, P. M. Renzi, and L. C. Schneider. 1996. Hepatitis C virus infection associated with administration of intravenous immune globulin. A cohort study. *Journal of the American Medical Association* (Nov 20) 276(19):1563–7.

Brillanti, S., J. Garson, M. Foli, K. Whitby, R. Deaville, C. Masci, M. Miglioli, and L. Barbara. 1994. A pilot study of combination therapy with ribavirin plus interferon alfa for interferon alfa-resistant chronic hepatitis C. *Gastroenterology* (Sep) 107(3):812–7.

Bruix, J. 1997. Treatment of hepatocellular carcinoma. *Hepatology* 25:259–62.

Buscarini, L., M. Di Stasi, E. Buscarini, F. Fornari, L. Squassante, S. Rossi, and M. Silva. 1996. Clinical presentation, diagnostic work-up, and therapeutic choices in two consecutive series of patients with hepatocellular carcinoma. *Oncology* (May-Jun) 53(3):204–9.

Caldwell, S. H., L. J. Jeffers, A. Ditomaso, A. Millar, R. M. Clark, A. Rabassa, K. R. Reddy, M. De Medina, and E. R. Schiff. 1991. Antibody to hepatitis C is common among patients with alcoholic liver disease with and without risk factors. *American Journal of Gastroenterology* (Sep) 86(9):1219–23.

Calleja, J. L., A. Albillos, G. Cacho, J. Iborra, L. Abreu, and P. Escartin. 1996. Interferon and prednisone therapy in chronic hepatitis C with non-organ-specific antibodies. *Journal of Hepatology* (Mar) 24(3):308–12.

Camarero, C., I. Martos, R. Delgado, L. Suarez, H. Escobar, and M. Mateos. 1993. Horizontal transmission of hepatitis C virus in households of infected children. *Journal of Pediatrics* (Jul) 123(1):98–9.

Camps, J., N. Garcia, J. I. Riezu-Boj, M. P. Civeira, and J. Prieto. 1993. Ribavirin in the treatment of chronic hepatitis C unresponsive to alfa interferon. *Journal of Hepatology* (Nov) 19(3):408–12.

Camps, J., M. Garcia-Granero, J. I. Riezu-Boj, E. Larrea, E. de Alava, M. P. Civeira, A. Castilla, and J. Prieto. 1994. Prediction of sustained remission of chronic hepatitis C after a 12-month course of alfa interferon. *Journal of Hepatology* (Jul) 21(1):4–11.

Carithers, R. L. 1997. Therapy of hepatitis C: interferon alfa-2b. *NIH Consensus Development Conference on Management of Hepatitis C* (Mar).

Casanova, R. L., and N. Gitlin. 1995. Treatments for hepatitis C: refinements in the recipe? *American Journal of Gastroenterology* (Nov) 90(11):2065–6.

Caselmann, W. H., and M. Alt. 1996. Hepatitis C virus infection as a major risk factor for hepatocellular carcinoma. *Journal of Hepatology* 24(2 Suppl):61–6.

Castells, L., V. Vargas, A. Gonzalez, J. Esteban, R. Esteban, and J. Guardia. 1995. Long interval between HCV infection and development of hepatocellular carcinoma. *Liver* (Jun) 15(3):159–63.

CDC Prevention Guidelines. 1997. Hepatitis C Prevention. CDC online.

Chan, T. M., A. S. Lok, I. K. Cheng, and R. T. Chan. 1993. Prevalence of hepatitis C virus infection in hemodialysis patients: a longitudinal study comparing the results of RNA and antibody assays. *Hepatology* (Jan) 17(1):5–8. Comment in: *Hepatology* 1994 (Apr) 19(4):1061.

Chan, T. M., A. S. Lok, I. K. Cheng, and R. T. Chan. 1993. A prospective study of hepatitis C virus infection among renal transplant recipients. *Gastroenterology* (Mar) 104(3):862–8.

Chayama, K., M. Kobayashi, A. Tsubota, I. Koida, Y. Arase, S. Saitoh, K. Ikeda, and H. Kumada. 1995. Molecular analysis of intraspousal transmission of hepatitis C virus. *Journal of Hepatology* (Apr) 22(4):431–9.

Chazouilleres, O., and T. L. Wright. 1995. Hepatitis C and liver transplantation. *Journal of Gastroenterology and Hepatology* (Jul-Aug) 10(4):471–80.

Chemello, L., D. Cavalletto, P. Pontisso, F. Bortolotti, C. Donada, V. Donadon, M. Frezza, P. Casarin, and A. Alberti. 1993. Patterns of antibodies to hepatitis C virus in patients with chronic non-A, non-B hepatitis and their relationship to viral replication and liver disease. *Hepatology* (Feb) 17(2):179–82.

Chemello, L., L. Cavalletto, F. Noventa, P. Bonetti, C. Casarin, E. Bernardinello, P. Pontisso, C. Donada, P. Casarin, F. Belussi, et al. 1995. Predictors of sustained response, relapse and no response in patients with chronic hepatitis C treated with interferon-alpha. *Journal of Viral Hepatology* 2(2):91–6.

Chetwynd, J. 1997. The time bomb of hepatitis C. *U.S. News & World Report* (Apr 7) 122(13):37.

Chiaramonte, M., T. Stroffolini, U. Lorenzoni, F. Minniti, S. Conti, A. Floreani, E. Ntakirutimana, A. Vian, T. Ngatchu, and R. Naccarato. 1996. Risk factors in community-acquired chronic hepatitis C virus infection: a case-control study in Italy. *Journal of Hepatology* (Feb) 24(2):129–34.

Chiba, T., Y. Matsuzaki, M. Abei, et al. 1996. The role of previous hepatitis B virus infection and heavy smoking in hepatitis C virus–related hepatocellular carcinoma. *American Journal of Gastroenterology* 91:119–203.

Chiba, T., Y. Matsuzaki, M. Abei, J. Shoda, T. Aikawa, N. Tanaka, and T. Osuga. 1996. Multivariate analysis of risk factors for hepatocellular carcinoma in patients with hepatitis C virus–related liver cirrhosis. *Journal of Gastroenterology* (Aug) 31(4):552–8.

Choo, Q. L., G. Kuo, A. J. Weiner, L. R. Overby, D. W. Bradley, and M. Houghton. 1989. Isolation of a cDNA clone derived from a blood-borne non-A, non-B viral hepatitis genome. *Science* 244:359–62.

Chu, C. M., I. S. Sheen, and Y. F. Liaw. 1994. The role of hepatitis C virus in fulminant viral hepatitis in an area with endemic hepatitis A and B. *Gastroenterology* (Jul) 107(1):189–95.

Clifford, B. D., D. Donahue, L. Smith, E. Cable, B. Luttig, M. Manns, and H. L. Bonkovsky. 1995. High prevalence of sero-logical markers of autoimmunity in patients with chronic hepatitis C. *Hepatology* (Mar) 21(3):613–9.

Colombo, M., Q. L. Choo, E. Del Ninno, et al. 1989. Prevalence of antibodies to hepatitis C virus in Italian patients with hepato-cellular carcinoma. *Lancet* 2:100–8.

Coltorti, M., N. Caporaso, F. Morisco, R. Suozzo, M. Romano, and M. D'Antonio. 1994. Prevalence of hepatitis C virus infection in the household contacts of patients with HCV-related chronic liver disease. *Infection* (May-Jun) 22(3):183–6.

Conrad, M. E. 1988. Prevention of post-transfusion hepatitis. *Lancet* 339(2):217.

Conry-Cantilena, C., M. A. Vanraden, J. Gibble, et al. 1996. Routes of infection, viremia, and liver disease in blood donors found to have hepatitis C infection. *New England Journal of Medicine* 334:1691–6.

Couzigou, P., L. Richard, F. Dumas, L. Schouler, and H. Fleury. 1993. Detection of HCV-RNA in saliva of patients with chronic hepatitis C. *Gut* 34(2 Suppl):S59–60.

Coverdale, S., K. Byth, J. Field, C. Liddle, R. Lin, and G. C. Farrell. 1995. Antipyrine clearance and response to interferon treatment in patients with chronic active hepatitis C. *Hepatology* (Oct) 22(4 Pt 1):1065–71.

Craxi, A., P. Almasio, and S. Schalm. 1996. Evaluation of efficacy of antiviral therapy for chronic hepatitis C: a EUROHEP Consensus Report on response criteria. *Journal of Viral Hepatology* (Sep) 3(5):273–6.

Curley, S. A., F. Izzo, A. Gallipoli, M. de Bellis, F. Cremona, and V. Parisi. 1995. Identification and screening of 416 patients with chronic hepatitis at high risk to develop hepatocellular cancer. *Annals of Surgery* (Sep) 222(3):375–80; discussion 380–3.

Daikos, G. L., S. Lai, and M. A. Fischl. 1994. Hepatitis C virus infection in a sexually active inner city population. The potential for heterosexual transmission. *Infection* (Mar-Apr) 22(2):72–6.

Davis, G. L. Hepatitis C virus infection among health care workers. 1996. *Journal of the American Medical Association* (May 15) 275(19):1474.

———. 1997. Predictive factors for a beneficial response. *NIH Consensus Development Conference on Management of Hepatitis C* (Mar).

Davis, G. L., and J. Y. Lau. 1995. Choice of appropriate end points of response to interferon therapy in chronic hepatitis C virus infection. *Journal of Hepatology* 22(1 Suppl):110–4.

Desmet, V. J., M. Gerber, J. H. Hoofnagle, M. Manns, and P. J. Scheuer. 1994. Classification of chronic hepatitis: diagnosis, grading, and staging. *Hepatology* 19:1513–20.

Diago, M., R. Zapater, C. Tuset, P. Carbonell, C. Gonzalez, R. Cors, and E. Casas. 1996. Intrafamily transmission of hepatitis C virus: sexual and non-sexual contacts. *Journal of Hepatology* (Aug) 25(2):125–8.

Diamantis, I. D., C. E. McGandy, T. J. Chen, Y. F. Liaw, F. Gudat, and L. Bianchi. 1994. Detection of hepatitis B and C viruses in liver tissue with hepatocellular carcinoma. *Journal of Hepatology* (Mar) 20(3):405–9.

Di Bisceglie, A. M. 1997. Hepatitis C and hepatocellular carcinoma. *NIH Consensus Development Conference on Management of Hepatitis C* (Mar).

———. 1995. Liver transplantation for hepatitis C: the promise and the challenge [editorial]. *Hepatology* (Aug) 22(2):660–2.

Di Bisceglie, A. M., B. R. Bacon, D. E. Kleiner, and J. H. Hoofnagle. 1994. Increase in hepatic iron stores following prolonged therapy with ribavirin in patients with chronic hepatitis C. *Journal of Hepatology* (Dec) 21(6):1109–12.

Di Bisceglie, A. M., H. S. Conjeevaram, M. W. Fried, R. Sallie, Y. Park, C. Yurdaydin, M. Swain, D. E. Kleiner, K. Mahaney, and J. H. Hoofnagle. 1995. Ribavirin as therapy for chronic hepatitis C. A randomized, double-blind, placebo-controlled trial. *Annals of Internal Medicine* (Dec 15) 123(12):897–903.

Di Bisceglie, A. M., P. Martin, C. Kassianides, M. Lisker-Melman, L. Murray, J. Waggoner, Z. Goodman, S. M. Banks, and J. H. Hoofnagle. 1989. Recombinant interferon alfa therapy for chronic hepatitis C. A randomized, double-blind, placebo-controlled trial. *New England Journal of Medicine* (Nov 30) 321(22):1506–10.

Di Bisceglie, A. M., S. E. Order, J. L. Klein, et al. 1991. The role of chronic viral hepatitis in hepatocellular carcinoma in the U.S. *American Journal of Gastroenterology* 86:335–8.

Di Bisceglie, A. M., M. Shindo, T. L. Fong, M. W. Fried, M. G. Swain, N. V. Bergasa, C. A. Axiotis, J. G. Waggoner, Y. Park, and J. H. Hoofnagle. 1992. A pilot study of ribavirin therapy for chronic hepatitis C. *Hepatology* (Sep) 16(3):649–54.

Di Bisceglie, A. M., L. H. Simpson, M.T. Lotze, et al. 1994. Development of hepatocellular carcinoma among patients with chronic liver disease due to hepatitis C viral infection. *Journal of Clinical Gastroenterology* 19:222–6.

Dienstag, J. L. 1997. The natural history of chronic hepatitis C and what we should do about it [editorial]. *Gastroenterology* (Feb) 25(2):651–5.

Dolan, P. J., R. M. Skibba, R. C. Hagan, and W. R. Kilgore. 1991. Hepatitis C: prevention and treatment. *American Family Physician* (Apr) 43(4):1347–50, 1355–60.

Dourakis, S. P., M. Deutsch, and S. J. Hadziyannis. 1996. Immune thrombocytopenia and alpha-interferon therapy. *Journal of Hepatology* (Dec) 25(6):972–5.

Dusheiko, G. 1997. Side effects of interferon alpha in viral hepatitis. *NIH Consensus Development Conference on Management of Hepatitis C* (Mar).

Dusheiko, G. M., S. Khakoo, P. Soni, and L. Grellier. 1996. A rational approach to the management of hepatitis C infection. *British Medical Journal* (Feb 10) 312(7027):357–64.

Dusheiko, G., J. Main, H. Thomas, O. Reichard, C. Lee, et al. 1996. Ribavirin treatment for patients with chronic hepatitis C: results of a placebo-controlled study. *Journal of Hepatology* (Nov) 25(5):591–8.

Dusheiko, G., and P. Simmonds. 1994. Sequence variability of hepatitis C virus and its clinical relevance. *Journal of Viral Hepatitis* 1:3–15.

Dussol, B., P. Berthezene, P. Brunet, C. Roubicek, and Y. Berland. 1995. Hepatitis C virus infection among chronic dialysis patients in the south of France: a collaborative study. *American Journal of Kidney Disease* (Mar) 25(3):399–404.

Ellett, H., and M. L. Shiffman. 1993. Natural history of post-transfusion hepatitis: the wolf in sheep's clothing. *American Journal of Gastroenterology* (Nov) 88(11):1970–2.

Enomoto, N., I. Sakuma, Y. Asahina, M. Kurosaki, T. Murakami, C. Yamamoto, Y. Ogura, N. Izumi, F. Marumo, and C. Sato. 1996. Mutations in the nonstructural protein 5A gene and response to interferon in patients with chronic hepatitis C virus 1b infection. *New England Journal of Medicine* (Jan 11) 334(2):77–81.

Esteban, J. I., J. Gomez, M. Martell, B. Cabot, J. Quer, J. Camps, A. Gonzalez, T. Otero, A. Moya, R. Esteban, et al. 1996. Transmission of hepatitis C virus by a cardiac surgeon. *New England Journal of Medicine* (Feb 29) 334(9):555–60.

Everhart, J. E., A. M. Di Bisceglie, L. M. Murray, et al. 1990. Risk for non-A, non-B (type C) hepatitis through sexual or household contact with chronic carriers. *Annals of Internal Medicine* 112:544–5.

Fackelmann, K. A. 1994. Changing hepatitis C evades immune system (new vaccines needed). *Science News* 146(6):85.

Farci, P., H. J. Alter, S. Govindarajan, et al. 1992. Lack of protective immunity against reinfection with hepatitis C virus. *Science* 258:135–40.

Farci P., H. J. Alter, A. Shimoda, S. Govindarajan, L. C. Cheung, J. C. Melpolder, R. A. Sacher, J. W. Shih, and R. H. Purcell. 1996.

Hepatitis C virus-associated fulminant hepatic failure. *New England Journal of Medicine* (Aug 29) 335(9):631–4.

Farci, P., H. J. Alter, D. Wong, et al. 1991. A long-term study of hepatitis C virus replication in non-A non-B hepatitis. *New England Journal of Medicine* 325:98–104.

Farrell, G. 1997. Interferon alfa-n 1 trials. *NIH Consensus Development Conference on Management of Hepatitis C* (Mar).

Fattovich, G., G. Giustina, F. Degos, et al. 1997. Morbidity and mortality in compensated cirrhosis type C: a retrospective follow-up study of 384 patients. *Gastroenterology* 112:463–72.

Fattovich, G., G. Giustina, S. Favarato, and A. Ruol. 1996. A survey of adverse events in 11,241 patients with chronic viral hepatitis treated with alfa interferon. *Journal of Hepatology* (Jan) 24(1):38–47.

Feray, C., M. Gigou, D. Samuel, V. Paradis, et al. 1994. The course of hepatitis C virus infection after liver transplantation. *Hepatology* 20:1137–43.

Feray, C., D. Samuel, M. Gigou, V. Paradis, M. F. David, C. Lemonnier, M. Reynes, and H. Bismuth. 1995. An open trial of interferon alfa recombinant for hepatitis C after liver transplantation: antiviral effects and risk of rejection. *Hepatology* (Oct) 22(4 Pt 1):1084–9.

Ferenci, P. 1993. Historical treatment of chronic hepatitis B and chronic hepatitis C. *Gut* (1993) 34(2 Suppl):S69–73.

Feucht, H. H., B. Zollner, M. Schroter, H. Altrogge, and R. Laufs. 1995. Tear fluid of hepatitis C virus carriers could be infectious. *Journal of Clinical Microbiology* (Aug) 33(8):2202–3.

Fong, T. L., B. Valinluck, S. Govindarajan, F. Charboneau, R. H. Adkins, and A. G. Redeker. 1994. Short-term prednisone therapy affects aminotransferase activity and hepatitis C virus

RNA levels in chronic hepatitis C. *Gastroenterology* (Jul) 107(1):196–9.

Galeazzi, B., A. Tufano, E. Barbierato, and F. Bortolotti. 1995. Hepatitis C virus infection in Italian intravenous drug users: epidemiological and clinical aspects. *Liver* (Aug) 15(4):209–12.

Gane, E. J., N. V. Naoumov, K. P. Qian, M. U. Mondelli, G. Maertens, B. C. Portmann, J. Y. Lau, and R. Williams. 1996. A longitudinal analysis of hepatitis C virus replication following liver transplantation. *Gastroenterology* (Jan) 110(1):167–77.

Gane, E. J., B. C. Portmann, N. V. Naoumov, H. M. Smith, J. A. Underhill, P. T. Donaldson, G. Maertens, and R. Williams. 1996. Long-term outcome of hepatitis C infection after liver transplantation. *New England Journal of Medicine* (Mar 28) 334(13):815–20.

Garfein, R. S., D. Vlahov, N. Galai, M. C. Doherty, and K. E. Nelson. 1996. Viral infections in short-term injection drug users: the prevalence of the hepatitis C, hepatitis B, human immunodeficiency, and human T-lymphotropic viruses. *American Journal of Public Health* (May) 86(5):655–61.

Gerberding, J. L. 1994. Incidence and prevalence of human immunodeficiency virus, hepatitis B virus, hepatitis C virus, and cytomegalovirus among health care personnel at risk for blood exposure: final report from a longitudinal study. *Journal of Infectious Disease* (Dec) 170(6):1410–7.

Gibas, A. L. 1993. Use of interferon in the treatment of chronic viral hepatitis. *Gastroenterologist* (Jun) 1(2):129–42.

Goritsas, C. P., A. Athanasiadou, A. Arvaniti, and C. Lampropoulou-Karatza. 1995. The leading role of hepatitis B and C viruses as risk factors for the development of hepatocellular carcinoma. A case control study. *Journal of Clinical Gastroenterology* (Apr) 20(3):220–4.

Gretch, D. 1997. Diagnostic Tests for Hepatitis C. *NIH Consensus Development Conference on Management of Hepatitis C* (March).

Gretch, D. R., C. E. Bacchi, L. Corey, C. dela Rosa, R. R. Lesniewski, K. Kowdley, A. Gown, I. Frank, J. D. Perkins, and R. L. Carithers, Jr. 1995. Persistent hepatitis C virus infection after liver transplantation: clinical and virological features. *Hepatology* (Jul) 22(1):1–9.

Gretch, D., I. Corey, J. Wilson, et al. 1994. Assessment of hepatitis C virus RNA levels by quantitative competitive RNA polymerase chain reaction: high-titer viremia correlates with advanced stage of disease. *Journal of Infectious Disease* 169:1219–25.

Griffith, H. 1995. *Complete Guide to Symptoms, Illness, and Surgery.* New York: The Body Press/Perigee Books.

Grimm, I., and N. Shaheen. 1996. Can interferon prevent hepatocellular carcinoma in hepatitis C virus-induced cirrhosis? *Gastroenterology* (Jun) 110(6):2019–21.

Gurakar, A., S. Fagiuoli, H. Faruki, N. De Maria, M. Balkan, D. H. Van Thiel, and L. Friedlander. 1995. Utility of hepatitis C virus RNA determinations in hepatic tissue as an end point for interferon treatment of chronic hepatitis C. *Hepatology* (Oct) 22(4 Pt 1):1109–12.

Hammel, P., P. Marcellin, M. Martinot-Peignoux, B. N. Pham, C. Degott, R. Level, V. Lefort, A. Benhallem, S. Erlinger, and J. P. Benhamou. 1994. Etiology of chronic hepatitis in France: predominant role of hepatitis C virus. *Journal of Hepatology* (Oct) 21(4):618–23.

Hanada, H., K. Hino, K. Fujii, M. Okazaki, and K. Okita. 1995. Rebound phenomenon of hepatitis C viremia after interferon therapy in relapsed patients with chronic hepatitis C. *Journal of Gastroenterology* (Jun) 30(3):347–50.

Harper, S. E., and J. L. Dienstag. 1996. Can interferon alfa treatment prevent hepatocellular carcinoma in patients with chronic hepatitis C infection and compensated cirrhosis? *Hepatology* (Apr) 23(4):930–3.

Haruna, Y., N. Hayashi, T. Kamada, P. Hytiroglou, S. N. Thung, and M. A. Gerber. 1994. Expression of hepatitis C virus in hepatocellular carcinoma. *Cancer* (May 1) 73(9):2253–8.

Hasan, F., L. J. Jeffers, M. De Medina, K. R. Reddy, T. Parker, E. R. Schiff, M. Houghton, Q. L. Choo, and G. Kuo. 1990. Hepatitis C-associated hepatocellular carcinoma. *Hepatology* (Sep) 12(3 Pt 1):589–91.

Hayashi, J., M. Ohmiya, Y. Kishihara, Y. Tani, N. Kinukawa, H. Ikematsu, and S. Kashiwagi. 1994. A statistical analysis of predictive factors of response to human lymphoblastoid interferon in patients with chronic hepatitis C. *American Journal of Gastroenterology* (Dec) 89(12):2151–6.

Health and Human Services, U.S. 1993. "Hepatitis C Prevention," pamphlet by the U.S. Dept. of Health and Human Services (Apr).

Hiramatsu, N., N. Hayashi, A. Kasahara, H. Hagiwara, T. Takehara, Y. Haruna, M. Naito, H. Fusamoto, and T. Kamada. 1995. Improvement of liver fibrosis in chronic hepatitis C patients treated with natural interferon alpha. *Journal of Hepatology* (Feb) 22(2):135–42.

Hollinger, F. B., and H. J. Lin. 1992. Community-acquired hepatitis C virus infection [editorial]. *Gastroenterology* (Apr) 102(4 Pt 1):1426–9.

Honda, M., S. Kaneko, A. Sakai, et al. 1994. Degree of diversity of hepatitis C virus quasi species and progression of liver disease. *Hepatology* 20:1144–51.

Hoofnagle, J. H. 1997. Hepatitis C: the clinical spectrum of disease. *NIH Consensus Development Conference on Management of Hepatitis C* (Mar).

Hoofnagle, J. H., and A. M. Di Bisceglie. 1997. Drug therapy: the treatment of chronic viral hepatitis. *New England Journal of Medicine* (Jan 30) 336(5):347–56.

Hoofnagle, J. H., A. M. Di Bisceglie, and M. Shindo. 1993. Antiviral therapy of hepatitis C—present and future. *Journal of Hepatology* 17 (Suppl 3):S130–6.

Hoofnagle, J. H., and D. Lau. 1996. Chronic viral hepatitis—benefits of current therapies [editorial]. *New England Journal of Medicine* (May 30) 334(22):1470–1.

Hoofnagle, J. H., D. Lau, H. Conjeevaram, D. Kleiner, and A. M. Di Bisceglie. 1996. Prolonged therapy of chronic hepatitis C with ribavirin. *Journal of Viral Hepatology* (Sep) 3(5):247–52.

Hopf, U., B. Moller, D. Kuther, et al. 1990. Long-term follow up of post-transfusion and sporadic chronic hepatitis non-A, non-B frequency of circulating antibodies to hepatitis C virus. *Journal of Hepatology* 10:69–76.

Horiike, N., T. Masumoto, K. Michitaka, K. Kurose, S. M. Akbar, and M. Onji. 1996. Response to interferon in chronic hepatitis C due to mixed genotype infection. *Journal of Gastroenterology and Hepatology* (Apr) 11(4):353–7.

Horiike, N., T. Masumoto, K. Nakanishi, K. Michitaka, K. Kurose, I. Ohkura, and M. Onji. 1995. Interferon therapy for patients more than 60 years of age with chronic hepatitis C. *Journal of Gastroenterology and Hepatology* (May-Jun) 10(3):246–9.

Houghton, M. 1996. Hepatitis C virus. *Fields Virology.* 3rd ed. Philadelphia: Lippincott-Raven Publishers.

Houghton, M., A. Weiner, J. Han, et al. 1991. Molecular biology of the hepatitis C viruses: implications for diagnosis, development, and control of viral diseases. *Hepatology* 14:381–8.

Hsu, H. H., T. L. Wright, S. C. Tsao, C. Combs, M. Donets, S. M. Feinstone, and H. B. Greenberg. 1994. Antibody response to hepatitis C virus infection after liver transplantation. *American Journal of Gastroenterology* (Aug) 89(8):1169–74.

Hwang, S. J., M. J. Tong, P. P. Lai, E. S. Ko, R. L. Co, D. Chien, and G. Kuo. 1996. Evaluation of hepatitis B and C viral markers: clinical significance in Asian and Caucasian patients with hepatocellular carcinoma in the United States of America. *Journal of Gastroenterology and Hepatology* (Oct) 11(10):949–54.

Irie, Y., H. Hayashi, K. Yokozeki, T. Kashima, and K. Okuda. 1994. Hepatitis C infection unrelated to blood transfusion in hemodialysis patients. *Journal of Hepatology* (Apr) 20(4):557–9.

Ishibashi, M., H. Shinzawa, M. Kuboki, H. Tsuchida, and T. Takahashi. 1996. Prevalence of inhabitants with anti-hepatitis C virus antibody in an area following an acute hepatitis C epidemic: age- and area-related features. *Journal of Epidemiology* (Mar) 6(1):1–7.

Itoh, H., H. Nakata, Y. Yokoya, S. Nakashima, T. Yamanishi, T. Hara, J. Kawai, H. Miyamoto, K. Higashi, and S. Nishioka. 1996. Efficacy and side effects of intermittent recombinant interferon-alpha 2a in chronic aggressive hepatitis C: with or without initial daily administration. *Journal of Gastroenterology and Hepatology* (Aug)11(8):718–23.

Izzo, F., S. Curley, P. Maio, E. Leonardi, L. Imparato, S. Giglio, F. Cremona, and G. Castello. 1996. Correlation of soluble interleukin-2 receptor levels with severity of chronic hepatitis C virus liver injury and development of hepatocellular cancer. *Surgery* (Jul) 120(1):100–5.

Janssen, H. L., J. T. Brouwer, R. C. van der Mast, and S. W. Schalm. 1994. Suicide associated with alfa-interferon therapy for chronic viral hepatitis. *Journal of Hepatology* (Aug) 21(2):241–3.

Johnson, M. W., W. K. Washburn, R. B. Freeman, S. E. FitzMaurice, J. Dienstag, N. Basgoz, R. L. Jenkins, and A. B. Cosimi. 1996. Hepatitis C viral infection in liver transplantation. *Archives in Surgery* (Mar) 131(3):284–91.

Jouet, P., F. Roudot-Thoraval, D. Dhumeaux, et al. 1994. Comparative efficacy of interferon alfa in cirrhotic and noncirrhotic patients with non-A, non-B, C hepatitis. *Gastroenterology* 106:686–90.

Kanazawa, Y., N. Hayashi, E. Mita, T. Li, H. Hagiwara, A. Kasahara, H. Fusamoto, and T. Kamada. 1994. Influence of viral quasi-species on effectiveness of interferon therapy in chronic hepatitis C patients. *Hepatology* (Nov) 20(5):1121–30.

Kasahara, A., N. Hayashi, N. Hiramatsu, M. Oshita, H. Hagiwara, K. Katayama, M. Kato, M. Masuzawa, H. Yoshihara, Y. Kishida, et al. 1995. Ability of prolonged interferon treatment to suppress relapse after cessation of therapy in patients with chronic hepatitis C: a multicenter randomized controlled trial. *Hepatology* (Feb) 21(2):291–7.

Katkov, W. N., J. L. Dienstag, H. Cody, A. A. Evans, Q. L. Choo, M. Houghton, and G. Kuo. 1991. Role of hepatitis C virus in non-B chronic liver disease. *Archives in Internal Medicine* (Aug) 151(8):1548–52.

Kato, Y., K. Nakata, K. Omagari, R. Furukawa, Y. Kusumoto, I. Mori, H. Tajima, H. Tanioka, M. Yano, and S. Nagataki. 1994. Risk of hepatocellular carcinoma in patients with cirrhosis in Japan. Analysis of infectious hepatitis viruses. *Cancer* (Oct 15) 74(8):2234–8.

Kawano, T., M. Shigehira, H. Uto, T. Nakama, J. Kato, K. Hayashi, T. Maruyama, T. Kuribayashi, T. Chuman, T. Futami, and H. Tsubouchi. 1996. Retinal complications during interferon therapy for chronic hepatitis C. *American Journal of Gastroenterology* (Feb) 91(2):309–13.

Keefe, E. B., B. Hollinger, and Consensus Interferon Study Group. 1997. Consensus Interferon trials. *NIH Consensus Development Conference on Management of Hepatitis C* (Mar).

Kew, M. C., M. C. Yu, M. A. Kedda, A. Coppin, A. Sarkin, and J. Hodkinson. 1997. The relative roles of hepatitis B and C viruses in the etiology of hepatocellular carcinoma in southern African blacks. *Gastroenterology* (Jan) 112(1):184–7.

King, J. W. 1994. Hepatitis C virus. *Bug Bytes* (http://www.ccm.lsumc.edu/bugbytes/) 1:13 (Dec 27).

Kiyosawa, K., and S. Furuta. 1991. Review of hepatitis C in Japan. *Journal of Gastroenterology and Hepatology* (Jul-Aug) 6(4):383–91.

Kiyosawa, K., T. Sodeyama, E. Tanaka, et al. 1990. Interrelationship of blood transfusion, non-A, non-B hepatitis and hepatocellular carcinoma: analysis by detection of antibody to hepatitis C virus. *Hepatology* 12:671–5.

Kiyosawa, K., T. Sodeyama, E. Tanaka, Y. Nakano, S. Furuta, K. Nishioka, R. H. Purcell, and H. J. Alter. 1991. Hepatitis C in hospital employees with needlestick injuries. *Annals of Internal Medicine* (Sep 1) 115(5):367–9.

Kobayashi, M., E. Tanaka, E. Sodeyama, et al. 1996. The natural course of chronic hepatitis C: a comparison between patients with genotypes 1 and 2 hepatitis C viruses. *Hepatology* 23:695–9.

Kodama, T., S. Katabami, K. Kamijo, A. Katanuma, K. Yamashita, N. Azuma, T. Tamaki, and A. Yachi. 1994. Development of transient thyroid disease and reaction during treatment of chronic hepatitis C with interferon. *Journal of Gastroenterology* (Jun) 29(3):289–92.

Koff, R. S. 1991. Anti-HCV screening of blood donors: the impact in Spain. *Gastroenterology* (Mar) 100(3):839–41.

———. 1993. A redoubtable obstacle to a hepatitis C vaccine. *Gastroenterology* (Apr) 104(4):1228–9.

Kolata, G. 1995. The hepatitis scare: how serious is it? *Cosmopolitan* 218(1):168–71.

Koretz, R. L., H. Abbey, E. Coleman, and G. Gitnick. 1992. Non-A, non-B post-transfusion hepatitis: looking back in the second decade. *Annals of Internal Medicine* 16:273–81.

Koziel, M. J., and T. J. Liang. 1994. Vaccination against hepatitis C virus infection: miles to go before we sleep. *Hepatology* (Sep) 20(3):758–60.

Krawczynski, K., M. J. Alter, D. L. Tankersley, M. Beach, B. H. Robertson, S. Lambert, G. Kuo, J. E. Spelbring, E. Meeks, S. Sinha, and D. A. Carson. 1996. Effect of immune globulin on the prevention of experimental hepatitis C virus infection. *Journal of Infectious Disease* (Apr) 173(4):822–8.

Kroes, A. C., R. A. de Man, H. G. Niesters, S. W. Schalm, W. Weimar, and A. H. Balk. 1994. Fatal hepatitis C virus infection in a heart transplant recipient detectable by polymerase chain reaction only. *Journal of Hepatology* (Dec) 21(6):1113–5.

Kumada, T., S. Nakano, I. Takeda, K. Sugiyama, T. Osada, S. Kiriyama, Y. Sone, H. Toyoda, S. Shimada, M. Takahashi, and T. Sassa. 1997. Patterns of recurrence after initial treatment in patients with small hepatocellular carcinoma. *Hepatology* (Jan) 25(1):87–92.

Kumagai, N., S. Kuramochi, K. Toda, N. Iwabuchi, K. Tsuchimoto, S. Tsunematsu, H. Saito, T. Morizane, M. Tsuchiya, and H. Ishii. 1996. Assessment of histological features and outcome of interferon therapy in chronic hepatitis C. *Journal of Gastroenterology* (Feb) 31(1):69–74.

Lai, M. Y., J. H. Kao, P. M. Yang, J. T. Wang, P. J. Chen, K. W. Chan, J. S. Chu, and D. S. Chen. 1996. Long-term efficacy of ribavirin plus interferon alfa in the treatment of chronic hepatitis C. *Gastroenterology* (Nov) 111(5):1307–12.

Lam, J. P., F. McOmish, S. M. Burns, P. L. Yap, J. Y. Mok, and P. Simmonds. 1993. Infrequent vertical transmission of hepatitis C virus. *Journal of Infectious Disease* (Mar) 167(3):572–6.

Laskus, T., L. F. Wang, J. Rakela, H. Vargas, A. D. Pinna, A. C. Tsamandas, A. J. Demetris, and J. Fung. 1996. Dynamic behavior of hepatitis C virus in chronically infected patients receiving liver graft from infected donors. *Virology* (Jun 1) 220(1):171–6.

Lau, J. Y., G. L. Davis, M. E. Brunson, K. P. Qian, H. J. Lin, S. Quan, R. DiNello, A. J. Polito, and J. C. Scornik. 1993. Hepatitis C virus infection in kidney transplant recipients. *Hepatology* (Nov) 18(5):1027–31.

Lebovics, E., J. Lantin, G. Chaurushia, B. M. Dworkin, A. Casellas, and W. S. Rosenthal. 1995. The breakthrough phenomenon during alpha-interferon therapy of chronic hepatitis C: incidence, management, and outcome. *American Journal of Gastroenterology* (Jun) 90(6):951–4.

Lee, W. M. 1995. Mapping a strategy for curing hepatitis C. *Gastroenterology* (Mar) 108(3):945–6.

———. 1993. Should we transplant hepatitis C-positive organs? *Gastroenterology* (Jul) 105(1):300–2.

————. 1993. The silent epidemic of hepatitis C. *Gastroenterology* (Feb) 104(2):661–2.

————. 1997. Therapy of hepatitis C with interferon alpha-2a. *NIH Consensus Development Conference on Management of Hepatitis C* (Mar).

————. 1992. Where is the dividing line between autoimmune hepatitis and hepatitis C? *Gastroenterology* (May) 102(5):1814–5.

Lefkowitch, J. H., E. R. Schiff, G. L. Davis, R. P. Perrillo, K. Lindsay, H. C. Bodenheimer, Jr., L. A. Balart, T. J. Ortego, J. Payne, J. L. Dienstag, et al. 1993. Pathological diagnosis of chronic hepatitis C: a multicenter comparative study with chronic hepatitis B. The Hepatitis Interventional Therapy Group. *Gastroenterology* (Feb) 104(2):595–603.

Leikin, E. L., J. F. Reinus, E. Schmell, and N. Tejani. 1994. Epidemiologic predictors of hepatitis C virus infection in pregnant women. *Obstetrics and Gynecology* (Oct) 84(4):529–34.

Levrero, M., A. Tagger, C. Balsano, E. De Marzio, M. L. Avantaggiati, G. Natoli, D. Diop, E. Villa, G. Diodati, and A. Alberti. 1991. Antibodies to hepatitis C virus in patients with hepatocellular carcinoma. *Journal of Hepatology* (Jan) 12(1):60–3.

Liang, T. J., L. J. Jeffers, K. R. Reddy, M. De Medina, I. T. Parker, H. Cheinquer, V. Idrovo, A. Rabassa, and E. R. Schiff. 1993. Viral pathogenesis of hepatocellular carcinoma in the United States. *Hepatology* (Dec) 18(6):1326–33.

Liaw, Y. F., I. S. Sheen, S. M. Lin, T. J. Chen, and C. M. Chu. 1993. Effects of prednisolone pretreatment in interferon alfa therapy for patients with chronic non-A, non-B (C) hepatitis. *Liver* (Feb) 13(1):46–50.

Lin, H. H., J. H. Kao, H. Y. Hsu, Y. H. Ni, M. H. Chang, S. C. Huang, L. H. Hwang, P. J. Chen, and D. S. Chen. 1995. Absence of infection in breast-fed infants born to hepatitis C virus-infected mothers. *Journal of Pediatrics* (Apr) 126(4):589–91.

Lisker-Melman, M., A. M. Di Bisceglie, S. J. Usala, B. Weintraub, L. M. Murray, and J. H. Hoofnagle. 1992. Development of thyroid disease during therapy of chronic viral hepatitis with interferon alfa. *Gastroenterology* (Jun) 102(6):2155–60.

Lok, A., and N. T. Gunaratnam. 1997. Diagnosis of hepatitis C. *NIH Consensus Development Conference on Management of Hepatitis C* (Mar).

Marcellin, P. 1997. Treatment of patients with normal ALT levels. *NIH Consensus Development Conference on Management of Hepatitis C* (Mar).

Marranconi, F., P. Fabris, C. Stecca, L. Zampieri, M. C. Bettini, N. Di Fabrizio, and F. de Lalla. 1994. Prevalence of anti-HCV and risk factors for hepatitis C virus infection in healthy pregnant women. *Infection* (Sep-Oct) 22(5):333–7.

Martin, Justin. 1995. Hepatitis C, the quiet epidemic. *Fortune* 132(3):29–30.

Mattson, L., A. Sonnerborg, and O. Weiland. 1993. Outcome of acute symptomatic non-A, non-B hepatitis: a 13-year follow up study of hepatitis C virus markers. *Liver* 13:274–8.

Mazzaferro, V., E. Regalia, R. Doci, et al. 1996. Liver transplantation for the treatment of small hepatocellular carcinomas in patients with cirrhosis. *New England Journal of Medicine* 334:693–9.

Mazzella, G., E. Accogili, S. Sottili, et al. 1996. Alpha interferon treatment may prevent hepatocellular carcinoma in HCV-related liver cirrhosis. *Journal of Hepatology* 24:141–7.

Mele, A., L. Sagliocca, G. Manzillo, F. Converti, P. Amoroso, M. A. Stazi, L. Ferrigno, M. Rapicetta, E. Franco, B. Adamo, et al.

1994. Risk factors for acute non-A, non-B hepatitis and their relationship to antibodies for hepatitis C virus: a case-control study. *American Journal of Public Health* (Oct) 84(10):1640–3.

Minuk, G. Y. and B. G. Rosser. 1997. Counseling of patients with viral hepatitis. *Hepatitis Update #10 (on-line), Hepatitis Information Network* (May 3).

Misiani, R., P. Bellavita, D. Fenili, O. Vicari, D. Marchesi, P. L. Sironi, P. Zilio, A. Vernocchi, M. Massazza, G. Vendramin, et al. 1994. Interferon alfa-2a therapy in cryoglobulinemia associated with hepatitis C virus. *New England Journal of Medicine* (Mar 17) 330(11):751–6.

Muller, R. 1991. Interferons in chronic viral hepatitis. *Hepatogastroenterology* (Feb) 38(1):4–9.

———. 1996. The natural history of hepatitis C: clinical experiences. *Journal of Hepatology* 24(2 Suppl):52–4.

Munro, J., J. D. Briggs, and E. A. McCruden. 1996. Detection of a cluster of hepatitis C infections in a renal transplant unit by analysis of sequence variation of the NS5a gene. *Journal of Infectious Disease* (Jul) 174(1):177–80.

Murphy, E. L., S. Bryzman, A. E. Williams, H. Co-Chien, G. B. Schreiber, H. E. Ownby, R. O. Gilcher, S. H. Kleinman, L. Matijas, R. A. Thomson, and G. J. Nemo. 1996. Demographic determinants of hepatitis C virus seroprevalence among blood donors. *Journal of the American Medical Association* (Apr 3) 275(13):995–1000.

Naito, M., N. Hayashi, H. Hagiwara, N. Hiramatsu, A. Kasahara, H. Fusamoto, and T. Kamada. 1994. Serum hepatitis C virus RNA quantity and histological features of hepatitis C virus carriers with persistently normal ALT levels. *Hepatology* (Apr) 19(4):871–5.

Neal, K. R., J. Dornan, and W. L. Irving. 1997. Prevalence of hepatitis C antibodies among healthcare workers of two teaching hospitals. Who is at risk? *British Medical Journal* (Jan 18) 314(7075):179–80.

Nishiguchi, S., T. Juroki, S. Nakatani, H. Morimoto, et al. 1995. Randomised trial of effects of interferon-a on incidence of hepatocellular carcinoma in chronic active hepatitis C with cirrhosis. *Lancet* 346:1051–5.

Nishiguchi, S., T. Kuroki, T. Yabusako, S. Seki, K. Kobayashi, T. Monna, S. Otani, M. Sakurai, T. Shikata, and S. Yamamoto. 1991. Detection of hepatitis C virus antibodies and hepatitis C virus RNA in patients with alcoholic liver disease. *Hepatology* (Dec) 14(6):985–9.

Nishioka, K., J. Watanabe, S. Furuta, E. Tanaka, S. Lino, H. Suzuki, T. Tsuju, M. Yano, et al. 1991. A high prevalence of antibody to the hepatitis C virus in patients with hepatocellular carcinoma in Japan. *Cancer* 67:429–33.

Niu, M. T., M. J. Alter, C. Kristensen, and H. S. Margolis. 1992. Outbreak of hemodialysis-associated non-A, non-B hepatitis and correlation with antibody to hepatitis C virus. *American Journal of Kidney Disease* (Apr) 19(4):345–52.

Niu, M. T., P. J. Coleman, and M. J. Alter. 1993. Multicenter study of hepatitis C virus infection in chronic hemodialysis patients and hemodialysis center staff members. *American Journal of Kidney Disease* (Oct) 22(4):568–73.

Nompleggi, D. J., and H. Bonkovsky. 1997. Diet and chronic liver disease: an updated research report. American Liver Foundation report.

Nomura, A., G. N. Stemmermann, P. H. Chyou, and E. Tabor. 1996. Hepatitis B and C serologies among Japanese Americans with hepatocellular carcinoma. *Journal of Infectious Diseases* 173:1474–6.

Ohashi, K., M. Tsutsumi, Y. Nakajima, K. Kobitsu, H. Nakano, and Y. Konishi. 1996. Telomere changes in human hepatocellular carcinomas and hepatitis virus infected noncancerous livers. *Cancer* (Apr 15) 77(8 Suppl):1747–51.

Ohnishi, K., S. Matsuo, K. Matsutani, M. Itahashi, K. Kakihara, K. Suzuki, S. Ito, and K. Fujiwara. 1996. Interferon therapy for chronic hepatitis C in habitual drinkers: comparison with chronic hepatitis C in infrequent drinkers. *American Journal of Gastroenterology* (Jul) 91(7):1374–9.

Ohto, H., S. Terazawa, N. Sasaki, et al. 1994. Transmission of hepatitis C virus from mothers to infants. *New England Journal of Medicine* 330:744–50.

Okanoue, T., S. Sakamoto, Y. Itoh, M. Minami, K. Yasui, M. Sakamoto, K. Nishioji, T. Katagishi, Y. Nakagawa, H. Tada, Y. Sawa, M. Mizuno, K. Kagawa, and K. Kashima. 1996. Side effects of high-dose interferon therapy for chronic hepatitis C. *Journal of Hepatology* (Sep) 25(3):283–91.

Olynyk, J. K., K. R. Reddy, A. M. Di Bisceglie, L. J. Jeffers, T. I. Parker, J. L. Radick, E. R. Schiff, and B. R. Bacon. 1995. Hepatic iron concentration as a predictor of response to interferon alfa therapy in chronic hepatitis C. *Gastroenterology* (Apr) 108(4):1104–9.

Omata, M., and N. Kato. 1994. Recent advances in hepatitis C virus research. *Journal of Gastroenterology* (Jun) 29(3):377–82.

Oshita, M., N. Hayashi, A. Kasahara, H. Hagiwara, E. Mita, M. Naito, K. Katayama, H. Fusamoto, and T. Kamada. 1994. Increased serum hepatitis C virus RNA levels among alcoholic patients with chronic hepatitis C. *Hepatology* (Nov) 20(5):1115–20.

Osmond, D. H., N. S. Padian, H. W. Sheppard, S. Glass, S. C. Shiboski, and A. Reingold. 1993. Risk factors for hepatitis C virus seropositivity in heterosexual couples. *Journal of the American Medical Association* 269:361–5.

Ozyilkan, E. 1995. Chronic hepatitis C virus infection: clinical experience with 126 patients. *Journal of Chemotherapy* (Nov) 7 Suppl 4:206–7.

Paccagnini, S., N. Principi, E. Massironi, E. Tanzi, L. Romano, M. L. Muggiasca, M. C. Ragni, and L. Salvaggio. 1995. Perinatal transmission and manifestation of hepatitis C virus infection in a high risk population. *Journal of Pediatric Infectious Disease* (Mar) 14(3):195–9.

Pawlotsky, J. M., F. Roudot-Thoravel, M. Pellerin, et al. 1996. GBV-C infection in HCV-infected patients: epidemiological characteristics, influence on HCV infection, and response to interferon alfa therapy. *Hepatology* 24:226A.

Pereira, B. J., E. L. Milford, R. L. Kirkman, and A. S. Levey. 1991. Transmission of hepatitis C virus by organ transplantation. *New England Journal of Medicine* (Aug 15) 325(7):454–60.

Perrillo, R. P. 1997. Role of liver biopsy. *NIH Consensus Development Conference on Management of Hepatitis C.*

Polish, L. B., M. J. Tong, R. L. Co, et al. 1993. Risk factors for hepatitis C virus infection among health care personnel in a community hospital. *American Journal of Infection Control* 21:196–200.

Power, J. P., E. Lawlor, F. Davidson, et al. 1994. Hepatitis C viremia in recipients of Irish intravenous anti-D immunoglobulin. *Lancet* 344:1166–7.

Poynard, T., P. Bedossa, and P. Opolon. 1997. Natural history of liver fibrosis progression in patients with chronic hepatitis C. *Lancet* 349:825–32.

Poynard, T., V. Leroy, M. Cohard, T. Thevenot, P. Mathurin, P. Opolon, and J. P. Zarski. 1996. Meta-analysis of interferon randomized trials in the treatment of viral hepatitis C: effects of dose and duration. *Hepatology* (Oct) 24(4):778–89.

Preston, H., and T. L. Wright. 1996. Interferon therapy for hepatitis C. *Lancet* (Oct 12) 348(9033):973–4.

Purcell, R. H. 1993. The discovery of the hepatitis viruses. *Gastroenterology* (Apr) 104(4):955–63.

————. 1997. Hepatitis C virus: an introduction. *NIH Consensus Development Conference on Management of Hepatitis C.*

Rabinovitz, M., G. Block, and S. D. Finkelstein. 1996. Alpha-interferon retreatment of patients with chronic hepatitis C. *American Journal of Gastroenterology* (Aug) 91(8):1523–6.

Reichard, O., and O. Weiland. 1997. Ribavirin treatment alone or in combination with interferon. *NIH Consensus Development Conference on Management of Hepatitis C* (Mar).

Reinus, J. F., E. L. Leikin, H. J. Later, et al. 1992. Failure to detect vertical transmission of hepatitis C virus. *Annals of Internal Medicine* 17:881–6.

Roffi, L., G. C. Mels, G. Antonelli, G. Bellati, F. Panizzuti, A. Piperno, M. Pozzi, D. Ravizza, G. Angeli, F. Dianzani, et al. 1995. Breakthrough during recombinant interferon alfa therapy in patients with chronic hepatitis C virus infection: prevalence, etiology, and management. *Hepatology* (Mar) 21(3):645–9.

Romeo, R., S. Pol, P. Berthelot, C. Brechot. 1994. Eradication of hepatitis C virus RNA after alpha-interferon therapy. *Annals of Internal Medicine* (Aug 15) 121(4):276–7.

Romeo, R., M. A. Tommasinni, M. G. Rumi, et al. 1996. Genotypes in the progression of hepatitis C related cirrhosis and development of hepatocellular carcinoma. *Hepatology* 24:153A.

Rosenthal, P. 1993. Does maternal-neonatal transmission of hepatitis C occur—are we sure? *American Journal of Gastroenterology* (Aug) 88(8):1284–6.

Rosman, A. S., A. Waraich, K. Galvin, J. Casiano, F. Paronetto, and C. S. Lieber. 1996. Alcoholism is associated with hepatitis C but not hepatitis B in an urban population. *American Journal of Gastroenterology* (Mar) 91(3):498–505.

Rubin, R. A., M. Falestiny, and P. F. Malet. 1994. Chronic hepatitis C: advances in diagnostic testing and therapy. *Archives of Internal Medicine* (Feb 28) 154(4):387–92.

Rumi, M., E. Del Ninno, M. L. Parravicini, R. Romeo, R. Soffredini, M. F. Donato, J. Wilber, A. Russo, and M. Colombo. 1996. A prospective, randomized trial comparing lymphoblastoid to recombinant interferon alfa 2a as therapy for chronic hepatitis C. *Hepatology* (Dec) 24(6):1366–70.

Ryder, S. D., J. Koskinas, P. M. Rizzi, I. G. McFarlane, B. C. Portmann, N. V. Naoumov, and R. Williams. 1995. Hepatocellular carcinoma complicating autoimmune hepatitis: role of hepatitis C virus. *Hepatology* (Sep) 22(3):718–22.

Ryff, J. C. 1995. Usefulness of interferon for treatment of hepatitis C. *Journal of Hepatology* 22(1 Suppl):101–9.

Saez-Royuela, F., J. C. Porres, A. Moreno, I. Castillo, G. Martinez, F. Galiana, and V. Carreno. 1991. High doses of recombinant alpha-interferon or gamma-interferon for chronic hepatitis C: a randomized, controlled trial. *Hepatology* (Feb) 13(2):327–31.

Saito, T., H. Shinzawa, M. Kuboki, M. Ishibashi, H. Toda, Y. Okuyama, T. Nakamura, N. Yamada, H. Wakabayashi, H. Togashi, et al. 1994. A randomized, controlled trial of human lymphoblastoid interferon in patients with compensated type C cirrhosis. *American Journal of Gastroenterology* (May) 89(5):681–6.

Sallie, R. 1993. Is PCR a viable option for population screening? [news]. *Lancet* (Jun 19) 341(8860):1591–2.

Sanchez-Tapias, J. M., X. Forns, S. Ampurdanes, et al. 1996. Low dose alpha interferon therapy can be effective in chronic active hepatitis C. Results of a multicentre, randomised trial. *Gut* (Apr) 38(4):603–9.

Sanchez-Tapias, J. M., and J. Rodes. 1995. Dilemmas of organ transplantation from anti-HCV-positive donors. *Lancet* (Feb 25) 345(8948):469–70.

Saracco, G., and M. Rizzetto. 1997. A practical guide to the use of interferons in the management of hepatitis virus infections. *Drugs* (Jan) 53(1):74–85.

———. 1995. The long-term efficacy of interferon alfa in chronic hepatitis C patients: a critical review. *Journal of Gastroenterology and Hepatology* (Nov-Dec) 10(6):668–73.

Sata, M., K. Fukuizumi, Y. Uchimura, H. Nakano, K. Ishii, R. Kumashiro, M. Mizokami, J. Y. Lau, and K. Tanikawa. 1996. Hepatitis C virus infection in patients with clinically diagnosed alcoholic liver diseases. *Journal of Viral Hepatology* (May) 3(3):143–8.

Schalm, Solko. 1997. Treatment of patients with cirrhosis. *NIH Consensus Development Conference on Management of Hepatitis C.*

Schapiro, G. D., and L. S. Friedman. 1996. Autoimmune hepatitis and/or hepatitis C: how to decide. *Hepatology* (Mar) 23(3):647–9.

Schreiber, G. B., M. P. Busch, S. H. Kleinman, et al. 1996. The risk of transfusion-transmitted viral infections. *New England Journal of Medicine* 334:1685–90.

Science News. 1995. "Having the risk for hepatitis C?" *Science News* 147:11(171) (Mar 18).

Seeff, L. B. 1997. Natural history of hepatitis C. *NIH Consensus Development Conference on Management of Hepatitis C.*

———. 1997. Epidemiology and natural history of hepatitis C. *Hepatitis Information Network* (on-line) (June 17).

Seeff, L. B., Z. Buskell-Bales, E. C. Wright, et al. 1992. Long-term mortality after transfusion-associated non-A, non-B hepatitis. *New England Journal of Medicine* 327:1906–11.

Serfaty, L., P. Giral, A. Loria, T. Andreani, C. Legendre, and R. Poupon. 1994. Factors predictive of the response to interferon in patients with chronic hepatitis C. *Journal of Hepatology* (Jul) 21(1):12–7.

Seymour, C. A. 1996. Screening asymptomatic people at high risk for hepatitis C: the case for. *British Medical Journal* (May 25) 312(7042):1347–8.

Shakil, A. O., C. Conry-Cantilena, H. J. Alter, et al. 1995. Volunteer blood donors with antibody to hepatitis C virus: clinical, biochemical, virologic and histologic features. *Annals of Internal Medicine* 123:330–7.

Shakil, A. O., A. M. Di Bisceglie, and J. H. Hoofnagle. 1996. Seizures during alpha interferon therapy. *Journal of Hepatology* (Jan) 24(1):48–51.

Sharara, A. I., C. M. Hunt, and J. D. Hamilton. 1996. Hepatitis C. *Annals of Internal Medicine* (Oct 15) 125(8):658–68.

Sheen, I. S., Y. F. Liaw, D. Y. Lin, and C. M. Chu. 1996. Acute exacerbations in chronic hepatitis C: a clinicopathological and prognostic study. *Journal of Hepatology* (May) 24(5):525–31.

Sherlock, S. 1995. Antiviral therapy for chronic hepatitis C viral infection. *Journal of Hepatology* 23 Suppl 2:3–7.

Sherman, K. E., R. L. Creager, J. O'Brien, S. Sargent, S. Piacentini, and T. Thieme. 1994. The use of oral fluid for hepatitis C antibody screening. *American Journal of Gastroenterology* (Nov) 89(11):2025–7.

Shimizu, Y. K., S. M. Feinstone, M. Kohara, et al. 1996. Hepatitis C virus: detection of intracellular virus particles by electron microscope. *Hepatology* 23:205–9.

Shindo, M., K. Arai, Y. Sokawa, and T. Okuno. 1995. Hepatic hepatitis C virus RNA as a predictor of a long-term response to interferon-alfa therapy. *Annals of Internal Medicine* 122:586–91.

Sieck, J. O., M. E. Ellis, O. Alfurayh, M. A. Ali, H. A. Ali, A. Ayub, M. al-Fadda, M. Zafar, M. Halim, and S. S. Bernvil, et al. 1993. Histologically advanced chronic hepatitis C treated with recombinant alpha-interferon: a randomized, placebo-controlled, double-blind cross-over study. *Journal of Hepatology* (Nov) 19(3):418–23.

Silini, E., R. Bottelli, M. Asti, S. Bruno, et al. 1996. Hepatitis C virus genotypes and risk of hepatocellular carcinoma in cirrhosis: a case-control study. *Gastroenterology* 111:199–205.

Silva, A. E., B. Hosein, R. W. Boyle, C. T. Fang, M. Shindo, J. G. Waggoner, J. H. Hoofnagle, and A. M. Di Bisceglie. 1994. Diagnosis of chronic hepatitis C: comparison of immunoassays and the polymerase chain reaction. *American Journal of Gastroenterology* (Apr) 89(4):493–6.

Silverman, N. S., B. K. Jenkin, C. Wu, P. McGillen, and G. Knee. 1993. Hepatitis C virus in pregnancy: seroprevalence and risk factors for infection. *American Journal of Obstetrics and Gynecology* (Sep) 169(3):583–7.

Simmonds, P. 1995. Variability of hepatitis C virus. *Hepatology* (Feb) 21(2):570–83.

Simmonds, P., J. Mellor, A. Craxi, J. M. Sanchez-Tapias, A. Alberti, J. Prieto, M. Colombo, M. G. Rumi, O. Lo Iacano, S. Ampurdances-Mingall, X. Forns-Bernhardt, L. Chemello, M. P. Civeira, C. Frost, and G. Dusheiko. 1996. Epidemiological, clinical and therapeutic associations of hepatitis C types in western European patients. *Journal of Hepatology* (May) 24(5):517–24.

Simsek, H., C. Savas, H. Akkiz, and H. Telatar. 1996. Interferon-induced vitiligo in a patient with chronic viral hepatitis C infection. *Dermatology* 193(1):65–6.

Soni, P., G. M. Dusheiko, A. P. Dhillon, and T. J. Harrison. 1995. Genetic diversity of hepatitis C virus: implications for pathogenesis, treatment, and prevention. *Lancet* 345:562–3, (March 4).

Strassburg, C. P., and M. P. Manns. 1995. Autoimmune hepatitis versus viral hepatitis C. *Liver* (Oct) 15(5):225–32.

Takahashi, M., G. Yamada, and R. Miyamoto, et al. 1993. Natural course of chronic hepatitis C. *American Journal of Gastroenterology* 88:240–3.

Takano, S., Y. Ito, O. Yokosuka, M. Ohto, K. Uchiumi, K. Hirota, and M. Omata. 1994. A multicenter, randomized, controlled dose study of ursodeoxycholic acid for chronic hepatitis C. *Hepatology* (Sep) 20(3):558–64. Comment in: *Hepatology* (Sep) 22(3):1002.

Takano, S., K. Nakamura, S. Kawai, O. Yokosuka, Y. Satomura, and M. Omata. 1996. Prospective assessment of donor blood screening for antibody to hepatitis C virus by first- and second-generation assays as a means of preventing posttransfusion hepatitis. *Hepatology* (Apr) 23(4):708–12.

Takase, S., N. Takada, N. Enomoto, M. Yasuhara, and A. Takada. 1991. Different types of chronic hepatitis in alcoholic patients: does chronic hepatitis induced by alcohol exist? *Hepatology* (May) 13(5):876–81.

Tanaka, E., K. Kiyosawa, A. Matsumoto, T. Kashiwakuma, A. Hasegawa, H. Mori, O. Yanagihara, and Y. Ohta. 1996. Serum levels of hepatitis C virus core protein in patients with chronic hepatitis C treated with interferon alfa. *Hepatology* (Jun) 23(6):1330–3.

Tanaka, K., H. J. Alter, Y. Nakatsuki, et al. 1996. Effect of hepatitis G virus infection on chronic hepatitis C. *Annals of Internal Medicine* 125:740–3.

Tanaka, K., T. Hirohata, S. Koga, et al. 1991. Hepatitis C and hepatitis B in the etiology of hepatocellular carcinoma in the Japanese population. *Cancer Research* 51:2842–7.

Tanaka, K., K. Kiyosawa, T. Matsushima, et al. 1995. Epidemiology of genotypes of hepatitis C virus in Japanese patients with type C chronic liver disease: a multi-institution analysis. *Journal of Gastroenterology and Hepatology* 10:538–45.

Thomas, D. L., J. M. Zenilman, H. J. Alter, et al. 1994. Sexual transmission of hepatitis C virus among patients attending sexually transmitted disease clinics in Baltimore—an analysis of 309 sex partnerships. *Journal of Infectious Disease* 171:768–75.

Tibbs, C. J. 1995. Methods of transmission of hepatitis C. *Journal of Viral Hepatology* 2(3):113–9.

Tong, M. M., N. S. El-Farra, A. R. Reikes, and R. L. Co. 1995. Clinical outcomes after transfusion-associated hepatitis C. *New England Journal of Medicine* 332:1463–6.

Toyoda, H., S. Nakano, T. Kumada, I. Takeda, K. Sugiyama, T. Osada, and S. Kiriyama. 1996. Effect of daily administration period of natural alpha-interferon in patients with chronic hepatitis C. *American Journal of Gastroenterology* (Apr) 91(4):743–7.

Toyoda, H., S. Nakano, I. Takeda, T. Kumada, K. Sugiyama, T. Osada, S. Kiriyama, T. Suga, H. Ohki, O. Ito, et al. 1994. Re-treatment of chronic hepatitis C with interferon. *American Journal of Gastroenterology* (Sep) 89(9):1453–7.

Tremolada, F., C. Casarin, A. Alberti, et al. 1992. Non-A, non-B post-transfusion hepatitis: a 13-year follow-up study of hepatitis C virus markers. *Journal of Hepatology* 16:273–81.

Troisi, C. L., F. B. Hollinger, W. K. Hoots, C. Contant, J. Gill, M. Ragni, R. Parmley, C. Sexauer, E. Gomperts, G. Buchanan, et al. 1993. A multicenter study of viral hepatitis in a United States hemophiliac population. *Blood* (Jan 15) 81(2):412–8.

Tsubota, A., K. Chayama, Y. Arase, I. Koida, S. Saitoh, K. Ikeda, S. Iwasaki, T. Matsumoto, M. Kobayashi, and H. Kumada. 1993. Factors useful in predicting the response to interferon therapy in chronic hepatitis C. *Journal of Gastroenterology and Hepatology* (Nov-Dec) 8(6):535–9.

Tsubota, A., K. Chayama, K. Ikeda, A. Yasuji, I. Koida, S. Saitoh, M. Hashimoto, S. Iwasaki, M. Kobayashi, and K. Hiromitsu. 1994. Factors predictive of response to interferon-alpha therapy in hepatitis C virus infection. *Hepatology* (May) 19(5):1088–94.

Unoki, H., A. Moriyama, A. Tabaru, A. Masumoto, and M. Otsuki. 1996. Development of Sjogren's syndrome during treatment with recombinant human interferon-alpha-2b for chronic hepatitis C. *Journal of Gastroenterology* (Oct) 31(5):723–7.

Watanabe, U., E. Hashimoto, T. Hisamitsu, H. Obata, and N. Hayashi. 1994. The risk factor for development of thyroid disease during interferon-alpha therapy for chronic hepatitis C. *American Journal of Gastroenterology* (Mar) 89(3):399–403.

Weinstock, H. S., G. Bolan, A. L. Reingold, and L. B. Polish. 1993. Hepatitis C virus infection among patients attending a clinic for sexually transmitted diseases. *Journal of the American Medical Association* 269:392–4.

Yamada, G., M. Takatani, F. Kishi, M. Takahashi, T. Doi, T. Tsuji, S. Shin, M. Tanno, M. S. Urdea, and J. A. Kolberg. 1995. Efficacy of interferon alfa therapy in chronic hepatitis C patients depends primarily on hepatitis C virus RNA level. *Hepatology* (Nov) 22(5):1351–4.

Yamada, G., E. Tanaka, T. Miura, K. Kiyosawa, M. Yano, T. Matsushima, H. Tsubouchi, K. Ishikawa, M. Kohara, K. Hino, et al. 1995. Epidemiology of genotypes of hepatitis C virus in Japanese patients with type C chronic liver diseases: a multi-institution analysis. *Journal of Gastroenterology and Hepatology* (Sep-Oct) 10(5):538–45.

Yamakawa, Y., M. Sata, H. Suzuki, S. Noguchi, and K. Tanikawa. 1996. Higher elimination rate of hepatitis C virus among women. *Journal of Viral Hepatology* (Nov) 3(6):317–21.

Yamauchi, M., M. Nakahara, Y. Maezawa, S. Satoh, F. Nishikawa, M. Ohata, Y. Mizuhara, J. Hirakawa, H. Nakajima, K. Fujisawa, et al. 1993. Prevalence of hepatocellular carcinoma in patients with alcoholic cirrhosis and prior exposure to hepatitis C. *American Journal of Gastroenterology* (Jan) 88(1):39–43.

Yano, M., H. Kumada, M. Kage, K. Ikeda, K. Shimamatsu, O. Inoue, E. Hashimoto, J. H. Lefkowitch, J. Ludwig, and K. Okuda. 1996. The long-term pathological evolution of chronic hepatitis C. *Hepatology* (Jun) 23(6):1334–40.

Yotsuyanagi, H., K. Koike, K. Yasuda, K. Moriya, K. Hino, K. Kurokawa, and S. Iino. 1995. Hepatitis C virus genotypes and development of hepatocellular carcinoma. *Cancer* (Oct 15) 76(8):1352–5.

Yuki, N., N. Hayashi, A. Kasahara, H. Hagiwara, T. Takehara, M. Oshita, K. Katayama, H. Fusamoto, and T. Kamada. 1995. Pretreatment viral load and response to prolonged interferon-alpha course for chronic hepatitis C. *Journal of Hepatology* (Apr) 22(4):457–63.

Yun, Z. B., J. Odeberg, J. Lundeberg, O. Weiland, M. Uhlen, and A. Sonnerborg. 1996. Restriction of hepatitis C virus heterogeneity during prolonged interferon-alpha therapy in relation to changes in virus load. *Journal of Infectious Disease* (Apr) 173(4):992–6.

Zanetti, A. R., E. Tanzi, S. Paccagnin, N. Principi, et al. 1995. Mother-to-infant transmission of hepatitis C virus. *Lancet* 345:89–91.

Zein, N. N., J. Rakela, E. L. Krawitt, K. R. Reddy, T. Tominaga, D. H. Persing. 1996. Hepatitis C virus genotypes in the United States: epidemiology, pathogenicity, and response to interferon therapy. Collaborative Study Group. *Annals of Internal Medicine* (Oct 15) 125(8):634–9.

Zoli, M., D. Magalotti, G. Bianchi, C. Gueli, et al. 1996. Efficacy of a surveillance program for early detection of hepatocellular carcinoma. *Cancer* 78:977–85.

INDEX